Penelope Mary Fra
Editor

# Non-medical Prescribing in the United Kingdom

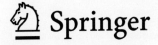 Springer

*Editor*
Penelope Mary Franklin
Honorary Associate Professor
Plymouth University
Executive Member of the
    Association for Prescribers
Essex
UK

ISBN 978-3-319-53323-0     ISBN 978-3-319-53324-7    (eBook)
DOI 10.1007/978-3-319-53324-7

Library of Congress Control Number: 2017946479

Printed on acid-free paper

This Springer imprint is published by Springer Nature
The registered company is Springer International Publishing AG
The registered company address is: Gewerbestrasse 11, 6330 Cham, Switzerland

# Foreword

I feel privileged to have been asked to write the foreword to this prestigious text. I say this because the book has been written by experts in the field of prescribing, both clinical and academic. It demonstrates a wealth of information enabling the reader to utilise this wisdom in order to supplement their practical knowledge in a manner that will assist towards competent prescribing.

This book is not only an aid to study but also can support the revalidation process of all health professionals who are prescribers.

In the UK, we have had legislation supporting prescribing for the last 18 years (since 1999), small steps initially, with a restricted formulary for district nurses and health visitors. By 2006, legislation was amended to enable access for non-medical prescribers to the whole of the British National Formulary. This was a seminal moment in terms of clinical practice in the UK as it provided an opportunity for health professionals other than nurses to be able to become prescribers. 18 years later, we have developed a robust body of evidence demonstrating that non-medical prescribing is beneficial for patients, cost effective and not duplicated. It has been demonstrated as equally effective as medical prescribing.

The most significant impact of non-medical prescribing has been patients receiving timely, expert and safe prescribing with increased access to medicines.

With an ever-increasing demand on healthcare, this text will provide further reference for the prescriber in their quest to increase their knowledge base and continue to push at professional practice boundaries, regardless of the discipline of the prescriber.

Colleagues across Europe and wider may also benefit from this text as a reference to what has been demonstrated as effective, safe practice when their countries' pioneers challenge the status quo of their health system.

I sincerely hope that you enjoy and find this text an aid to your learning and development.

Barbara Stuttle
Chair of The UK Association
for Nurse Prescribing
Rayleigh, UK

# Acknowledgement

Thank you to all who have made this book possible.

# Contents

1  **Introduction to Non-medical Prescribing:
   An Overview—Including Non-medical
   Prescribing in England**...................... 1
   Penny Franklin

**Part I  Non-medical Prescribing in Scotland,
         Wales and Northern Ireland**

2  **Non-medical Prescribing in Scotland**............ 17
   Andrew Rideout

3  **Non-medical Prescribing in Wales:
   Implementation and Governance**................ 33
   Eleri Mills

4  **Non-medical Prescribing in Northern Ireland** ..... 53
   F. Lloyd, C.G. Adair, J. Agnew, C. Blayney,
   G. Boyd-McMurtry, O. Brown, A. Campbell,
   K. Clarke, P. Crawford, D. Gill, C. Harrison,
   J. McClelland, M.F. McManus, M. McMullan,
   B. Moore, R. O'Hare, L. O'Loan, M. Tennyson,
   and H. Winning

**Part II  Non-medical Prescribing by Pharmacists
          and Allied Health Professionals**

5  **Non-medical Prescribing by Pharmacists** ......... 93
   Graham Brack

**6 Prescribing by Designated Allied Health Professionals: The AHP Experience** ............ 113
Alan Borthwick, Tim Kilmartin, Nicky Wilson, and Christina Freeman

**Part III The Practice, Art and Discipline(s) of Non-medical Prescribing**

**7 The Identity of Non-medical Prescribers** ........ 131
Sally Jarmain

**8 Non-medical Prescribing in Community Settings** .................................... 145
Sarah Kraszewski

**9 Prescribing for Long-Term Conditions** .......... 159
Helen Skinner

**10 Non-medical Prescribing in the Acute Setting** ....................................... 177
Jayne R. Worth

**11 Non-medical Prescribers Within Substance Misuse Services** ............................. 195
Hazel Roberts

**12 Non-medical Prescribing in Palliative and End-of-Life Care (EOLC)** ................. 215
Emma Sweeney

**Index** .......................................... 233

# List of Abbreviations

| | |
|---|---|
| AEI | Approved education institute |
| AHPs | Allied health professions/professionals |
| ANP | Advanced nurse practitioner |
| APP | Advanced pharmacy practice programme |
| AWMSG | All Wales medicines Strategy Group |
| AWTTC | All Wales Therapeutic and Toxicology Centre |
| BNF | British National Formulary |
| CDs | Controlled drugs |
| CMP | Clinical management plan |
| CNS | Clinical nurse specialist/s |
| COPD | Chronic obstructive pulmonary disease |
| CPD | Continuing professional development |
| CPNPs | Community practitioner nurse prescribers |
| CSP | Chartered Society of Physiotherapy |
| DEPs | Developing Eyecare Partnerships |
| DMP | Designated medical practitioner |
| DSMP | Designated supervising medical practitioner |
| EOLC | End of life care |
| ePACT | Electronic prescribing analysis and cost data |
| GB | Great Britain |
| GOC | General Optical Council |
| GP | General practitioner |
| GPhC | General Pharmaceutical Council |
| HAN | Hospital at night team |

| HCPC | Health and Care Professions Council |
|---|---|
| HD | High dependency (unit/care) |
| HSCB | Health Social Care Board (Northern Ireland) |
| HVs | Health visitors |
| ICU | Intensive care unit |
| IP/s | Independent prescriber/s |
| KSF | Knowledge and Skills Framework |
| LHB | Local Health Board |
| LTCs | Long-term conditions |
| MAI | Medication Appropriateness Index |
| MHRA | Medicines and Healthcare Products Regulatory Agency |
| MO | Medicines optimisation |
| MOQF | Medicines Optimisation Quality Framework |
| NAW | National Assembly for Wales |
| NHS | National Health Service |
| NI | Northern Ireland |
| NICE | National Institute for Health and Care Excellence |
| NICPLD | Northern Ireland Centre for Pharmacy Learning and Development |
| NIPEC | The Northern Ireland Practice and Education Council |
| NMC | Nursing and Midwifery Council |
| NMIPs | Non-medical independent prescribers |
| NMP | Non-medical prescribing |
| NPF | Nurse Prescribers' Formulary for Community Practitioners |
| NTA | The National Treatment Agency for Substance Misuse Services |
| PBP | Practice-based pharmacist/s |
| PCE | Pharmaceutical clinical effectiveness |
| PGD | Patient group direction |
| PIP | Pharmacist independent prescriber/ing |
| PSNI | Pharmaceutical Society of Northern Ireland |

| | |
|---|---|
| RPSGB | Royal Pharmaceutical Society of Great Britain |
| SCPHNs | Specialist community public health nurses |
| SP/s | Supplementary prescriber/s |
| SPM | Social photo matrix |
| TPN | Total parenteral nutrition |
| UK | United Kingdom |
| V100 | Community practitioner nurse prescriber with a specialist practice qualification (NMC annotation) |
| V150 | Community practitioner nurse prescriber without a specialist practice qualification (NMC annotation) |
| V200 | Extended formulary nurse prescriber (NMC annotation) |
| V300 | Nurse independent and supplementary prescriber (NMC annotation) |
| WeMeRec | Welsh Medicines Resource Centre |

All internet links were correct at time of going to press. However, it is acknowledged that these may go out of date and be revised, amended or removed from the relevant web sites.

# Chapter 1
# Introduction to Non-medical Prescribing: An Overview— Including Non-medical Prescribing in England

Penny Franklin

**Abstract** This book is intended for all innovators, policymakers and leaders who are considering implementing Non-medical Prescribing (NMP) both in the United Kingdom (UK) and further afield and, for practitioners who are working on the front line with patients. It covers historical perspective and current practice, with some pragmatic discussion and vision of where the practice of Non-medical Prescribing (NMP) might be going next. Contributors to the book discuss prescribing across the four divulged UK countries of Scotland, Wales, Northern Ireland and England. They have a range of academic, leadership and practice-based expertise and, are from the different professions representing some of the many and diverse disciplines where NMP is practised. There are many different fields of practice, and it would not be possible for the authors to represent all of these. It is up to the readers to take and transfer ideas and examples of good practice

P. Franklin
Executive Committee, Association for Prescribers,
Chelmsford, United Kingdom
e-mail: pfranklin@surrey.ac.uk

© Springer International Publishing AG 2017      1
P.M. Franklin (ed.), *Non-medical Prescribing in the United Kingdom*,
DOI 10.1007/978-3-319-53324-7_1

and policy making into their own areas using the scientific artistry and pragmatism that is needed in the world of health care today. What all of my co-authors share with you the reader is an enthusiasm for, and conviction of, the worth of NMP today, and ongoing into a changing world of health-care.

**Keywords** Non-medical Prescribing • Community Practitioner Nurse Prescribing • Independent Prescribing Supplementary Prescribing • Continuing professional development

## 1.1   Purpose of This Book

This book is designed for those who are thinking about how to take Non-medical Prescribing (NMP) forward in their area. NMP within the UK is now embedded in such a wide range of health-care professions and professional disciplines that it would be impossible within the remit of this book to cover them all. What you will find is a discussion of NMP and its differences in the four divulged countries that make up the UK (Scotland, Wales, Northern Ireland and England). There will be discussion of prescribing practice in the different professions that now have Non-medical Prescribing rights and commentary on prescribing in different areas by experts in disciplines including: community nursing, sexual health nursing, care of those with long-term conditions, drugs and alcohol dependency and end of life. There will be information about prescribing by nurses, midwives, pharmacists, podiatrists (chiropodists), physiotherapists, radiographers, dietitians and optometrists. There are many discipline-specific areas that practise NMP, and although it has not been possible to cover them all, it is hoped that readers will be able to take examples into their own areas. For those who are thinking of implementing prescribing within their area, policy and practice examples are threaded throughout. All authors illustrate innovative ways of thinking about the practice and implementation of NMP.

Authors showcase how NMP developed in their own areas in an often piecemeal fashion, sometimes in the face of opposition and at times against the odds. Chapters demonstrate how it is now embedded across professional health care, with vision of where we hope to go in the future. Authors are mindful that at the time of writing, the UK health-care system is set in a climate of austerity. However, we are ever enthusiastic about the difference that the practice of NMP has made to patients and professionals alike and are optimistic about future developments.

## 1.2   Historical Perspective

This section highlights the key changes to legislation that led to Non-medical Prescribing rights as they are today. It provides a brief overview of the different professions that can prescribe and of their rights. NMP rights have evolved differently within the four countries that make up the UK, and these will be discussed further on in the book.

Request for prescribing rights by Registered Nurses with a specialist community practice qualification (health visitors, district nurses and some practice nurses) formally started in 1986 with the publication of the Department of Health *Cumberlege Review of Neighbourhood Nursing*. Up to this time, the above groups of nurses had been recommending to doctors to prescribe for their patients, resulting in delay to patients obtaining medicines and putting doctors in the position of prescribing for patients who they had not assessed. The following 1989 Department of Health *Report of the Advisory Group on Nurse*

*Prescribing* led by Dr June Crown advised ministers in the UK of how the introduction of nurse prescribing could improve patient care.

Following amendments to the 1968 *Medicines Act* and the introduction in 1992 of *The Medicinal Products: Prescription by Nurses etc. Act*, the practice of nurse prescribing started. Piloting across two sites was rolled out nationally in 1994. Registered nurses with a specialist community practice qualification, having completed the required training at academic degree level, were able to prescribe from the limited *Nurse Prescribers' Formulary for Community Practitioners.* (NICE and BNF n.d.). It is of note that 2009 saw the introduction of Community Practitioner Nurse Prescribing for registered nurses and midwives without a specialist practice qualification (NMC 2009).

The success of the initial Community Practitioner Nurse Prescribing was noted, and the *Final Report on the Review of Prescribing, Supply and Administration of Medicines* in 1999 recommended that legal authority to prescribe should be extended to include new professional groups and, introduced the concepts of Independent and Dependent Prescriber (later to become Supplementary Prescriber). (see Table 1.1).

Registered nurses without a Community Specialist Practice qualification were granted prescribing rights as Extended Formulary Nurse Prescribers in 2002 (DoH 2002) which meant that they could prescribe within their scope of practice and competence from a limited range of drugs within the *British National Formulary (BNF)* in the areas of: minor illness, minor injury, health promotion and palliative care. The Extended Formulary for Nurse Prescribers is now obsolete.

Section 63 of the *Health and Social Care Act* 2001 permitted the introduction of Supplementary Prescribing (SP) for nurses and pharmacists (Table 1.1). In 2006, *the Medicines for Human Use (Prescribing) (Miscellaneous Amendments) Order and associated medicines regulations* enabled nurses and midwives

**Table 1.1** Illustrating the range of non-medical prescribing rights across the professions in England and the definitions of these rights

| Title | Legal status | Professions and qualification | Comments |
|---|---|---|---|
| Independent prescriber(s) (IP(s)) | Responsible and accountable for assessment, diagnosis and treatment (prescribing)—can prescribe within professional scope of practice and competence most drugs within the *British National Formulary*. | Medical Independent Prescribers are doctors and dentists who are subject to guidance from the General Medical Council. Available via: http://www.gmc-uk.org/guidance/ethical_guidance/14316.asp. Accessed 15 April 2017. Non-medical Independent Prescribers (NMIPs) are nurses, midwives pharmacists, physiotherapists, chiropodists/podiatrists, optometrists (from the Optometrists' Formulary) and therapeutic radiographers. All of whom who have successfully completed training at degree level or above and have been awarded their professional body recordable qualification as Non-medical Independent Prescriber. All are subject to standards and guidance from individual professional bodies. Available via: http://psnc.org.uk/dispensing-supply/receiving-a-prescription/who-can-prescribe-what/. Accessed 15 April 2017. | For Non-medical Prescribers, this training is now combined with Supplementary Prescribing. |

(continued)

**Table 1.1** (continued)

| Title | Legal status | Professions and qualification | Comments |
|---|---|---|---|
| Supplementary Prescriber(s) (SP(s)) | Prescribe in a voluntary partnership with Independent Medical Prescriber(s), with the agreement of the patient and using a patient-specific clinical management plan (CMP), that must be set up in advance of prescribing and preferably with the patient's agreement. Supplementary Prescribers can prescribe any drug from the *British National Formulary* (*BNF*) and within their professional scope of practice and competence. Supplementary Prescribers can prescribe schedules 2, 3 and 4 from the controlled drugs schedule (except diamorphine, cocaine and dipipanone for the treatment of addiction). | Includes nurses, midwives, pharmacists, physiotherapists, podiatrists (chiropodists), radiographers and dietitians who have successfully completed a period of training at degree level or above and have been awarded their professional body recordable qualification as Non-medical Supplementary Prescriber. | Nurses midwives, pharmacists, physiotherapists, podiatrists (chiropodists) and therapeutic radiographers now undertake a combined training as Independent and Supplementary Prescribers. Dietitians and diagnostic radiographers can train as Supplementary Prescribers only. |

| | | | |
|---|---|---|---|
| Non-medical Independent and Supplementary Prescribers | Can prescribe as both Independent and Supplementary Prescribers. There are profession-specific restrictions on who can prescribe what. Available via: https://psnc.org.uk/dispensing-supply/receiving-a-prescription/who-can-prescribe-what/. Accessed 15 April 2017. | Currently, nurses, midwives, pharmacists, physiotherapists, podiatrists (chiropodists) and therapeutic radiographers who have successfully completed a period of training at degree level or above and have been awarded their professional body recordable qualification as Non-medical Independent and Supplementary Prescriber. | Nurses, midwives, pharmacists, physiotherapists, podiatrists (chiropodists) and therapeutic radiographers now undertake a combined training as Independent and Supplementary Prescribers |
| Community Practitioner Nurse Prescribers | Prescribe from the *Nurse Prescribers' Formulary for Community Practitioners* only. Available via: https://www.evidence.nhs.uk/formulary/bnf/current/nurse-prescribers-formulary. Accessed 15 April 2017. | Includes nurses and midwives with the specialist community practice qualification of health visitor or district nurse, who have completed the training for the Nursing and Midwifery Council NMC V100 (NMC 2006) recordable qualification at degree level and above, and nurses without a specialist community practice qualification who have completed the training for the Nursing and Midwifery Council's recordable qualification of V150 Community Practitioner Prescriber (NMC 2009). | Can only prescribe from the *Nurse Prescribers' Formulary for Community Practitioners*. |

Who can prescribe what is profession specific; for a list please access following link. http://psnc.org.uk/dispensing-supply/receiving-a-prescription/who-can-prescribe-what/. Accessed 15 April 2017.

Prescribing rights for Non-medical Independent Prescribers are profession specific; a list of who can prescribe what is available via http://psnc.org.uk/dispensing-supply/receiving-a-prescription/who-can-prescribe-what/. Accessed 15 April 2017.

to train as Nurse and Midwife Independent Prescribers, meaning that they could prescribe *any licensed medicine (*i.e. *products with a valid marketing authorisation (licence) in the UK) including some controlled drugs, for any medical condition within their clinical competence* (DH 2006, pg. 3). Independent Prescribing (IP) for pharmacists was introduced at the same time. Pharmacist Independent Prescribers could not at this time, prescribe any controlled drugs (CDs). The biggest change was that Non-medical Independent Prescribers (NMIPs) carried the accountability for having assessed the patient, having made a diagnosis and ultimately for prescribing.

The above rapid changes to Nurse and Midwife Non-medical Prescribing led to the introduction of the Nursing and Midwifery Council's 2006 *Standards of Proficiency for Nurse and Midwife Prescribers* detailing both educational and practice standards for the above. The Health and Care Professions Council and the Royal Pharmaceutical Society introduced their standards in 2013, and the Royal College of Optometrists produced their own guidance for Independent Optometrist Prescribers Available via: https://psnc.org.uk/dispensing-supply/receiving-a-prescription/who-can-prescribe-what/. Accessed 15 April 2017.

Changes to the *Misuse of Drugs Regulations* in 2012 opened up the prescribing of CDs (except for diamorphine, cocaine and dipipanone for the treatment of addiction) to Nurse, Midwife and Pharmacist Independent Prescribers.

Registered physiotherapists, podiatrists and radiographers have been able to train as supplementary prescribers since 2005. Optometrists were also granted independent prescribing rights in 2008. General Optical Council Available at: https://www.optical.org/en/Education/Specialty_qualifications/independent-prescribing.cfm. Accessed 15 April 2015. Further changes in 2015 meant that registered physiotherapists, chiropodists/podiatrists and therapeutic radiographers could train as Independent Prescribers with profession-specific restrictions Available via: http://psnc.org.uk/dispensing-supply/receiving-a-prescription/

who-can-prescribe-what/. Accessed 15 April 2017. From 2016 dietitians could prescribe as Supplementary Prescribers only Available at: https://www.england.nhs.uk/ourwork/qual-clin-lead/ahp/med-project/dietitians/. Accessed 15 April 2015.

## 1.3   History Across the Four Countries

All of the above applies to Non-medical Prescribing in England. However, there are differences across the UK. Not only has Non-medical Prescribing evolved differently within the different professions, but also there have been differences in policy and implementation across the four countries, some of which will be discussed in the following chapters of this book. For example, in 2006 the Department of Health published a guide to implementing Nurse and Pharmacist prescribing within the National Health Service in England; however, this was not implemented in Wales. Other examples will be covered in following chapters.

## 1.4   Where We Are Now and Where We Are Going

Over the years, Non-medical Prescribing has evolved from Community Practitioner Nurse Prescribing (which still exists), through to the now obsolete Extended Formulary Nurse Prescribing, to Independent and Supplementary Prescribing for nurses, midwives, pharmacists, physiotherapists, podiatrists (chiropodists) and therapeutic radiographers. With some profession-specific restrictions (see Table 1.1), both IPs and SPs can prescribe within their scope of practice and professional competence from most of the *British National*

*Formulary*. Optometrists can prescribe as Independent Prescribers from the Optometrists' Formulary General Optical Council Available at: https://www.optical.org/en/Education/ Specialty_qualifications/independent-prescribing.cfm. Accessed 15 April 2015.

Non-medical Prescribing authority brings with it accountability and autonomy. This means that Non-medical Prescribers, all of whom are registered practitioners, now need to have advanced practice skills of consultation, assessment, diagnosis, communication and complex decision-making.

The delivery of health services in the UK is changing radically, and alongside of this, the need for Non-medical Prescribers is becoming mainstream. With more professions, for example, paramedics lobbying for prescribing rights, (https://www. rpharms.com/resources/frameworks/prescribers-competency-framework), it is likely that the practice will continue to grow to benefit patient care in other health-care registered professions.

## 1.5   Continuing Professional Development (CPD)

Non-medical Prescribing has reached maturity and is continuing to refine and develop. The Royal Pharmaceutical Society and the National Institute for Health and Care Excellence (NICE) jointly published the current *Competency Framework for All Prescribers* (RPS and NICE 2016). This new competency framework is centred on the domain of the patient with consultation and governance as the other two domains (RPS and NICE 2016). The framework is used as a benchmark for best practice by Medical and Non-medical Prescribers alike and demonstrates the level to which prescribing has become accepted and shared by the medical and allied health professions.

## 1.6 Training and Assessment

Currently, NMPs who are training are assessed in practice by Independent Medical Prescribers (doctors or dentists) in the role of Designated Medical Practitioners (DMPs). It can be argued that with 25 years of prescribing experience, the next step is for NMPs to gain autonomy by taking on the accountability for the assessment of NMPs. Although the above is controversial, it is debated within the discipline. However, it is important at this point that NMPs continue to acknowledge the immense expertise and support that is given by medical colleagues and there is a continuing need for joint sharing.

As already discussed, each professional body has its own set of standards governing the regulation and practice of their NMPs. The Nursing and Midwifery Council's standards have been in existence for over 10 years and are due to be updated in 2017.

The purpose of this book is to spark ideas for those who are starting out on the development of prescribing either in the UK or abroad and also to map our journey so far. The NMP journey has not always been straightforward. Authors in this book have been candid about some of the difficulties and pitfalls encountered along the way, as well as celebrating our successes. It is hoped that others will take what they need from our early faltering and now ever strengthening steps.

We are glad to share this journey with you and proud of where we have come from, where we now are and where we are going. It is up to you as a reader of this book to consider where you are and where you want to go next. As authors and experts in the field, we do not claim to have all of the answers; however, we are privileged to be able to share with you our passion for this most challenging and exciting discipline and hope that by demonstrating our learning, we can contribute to the ongoing journey of others.

# References

Department of Health (1989) Report of the advisory group on nurse prescribing. Department of Health, London

Department of Health (1999) Review of prescribing, supply and administration of medicines (The Crown Report). Available via http://webarchive.nationalarchives.gov.uk/+/www.dh.gov.uk/en/Publicationsandstatistics/Publications/PublicationsPolicyAndGuidance/DH_4077151. Accessed 10 Jun 2017

Department of Health (2002) Extending independent nurse prescribing within the NHS in England. Department of Health, London

Department of Health (2003) Supplementary prescribing. Available via http://webarchive.nationalarchives.gov.uk/+/www.dh.gov.uk/en/Healthcare/Medicinespharmacyandindustry/prescriptions/TheNon-MedicalPrescribingProgramme/supplementaryprescribing/DH_4123025. Accessed 10 Jun 2017

Department of Health (2006) Improving patients' access to medicines: a guide to implementing nurse and pharmacist independent prescribing within the NHS in England. Department of Health Gateway reference: 6429. Available via http://webarchive.nationalarchives.gov.uk/20130107105354/http:/www.dh.gov.uk/prod_consum_dh/groups/dh_digitalassets/@dh/@en/documents/digitalasset/dh_4133747.pdf. Accessed 10 Jun 2017

Department of Health and Social Security (1986) Neighbourhood nursing: a focus for care. Cumberlege report. HMSO, London

Health and Care Professions Council HCPC (2013) Standards for prescribing. Available via http://www.hcpc-uk.org/aboutregistration/standards/standardsforprescribing/. Accessed 29 Dec 2016

Health and Care Professions Council HCPC (2016) Available via http://www.hcpc-uk.co.uk/aboutregistration/medicinesandprescribing/. Accessed 15 April 2017

Health and Care Professions Council HCPC (n.d.) Available via http://www.hpc-uk.org/aboutregistration/medicinesandprescribing/. Accessed 30 Dec 2016

Health and Social Care Act (2001) Section 63 Chapter 15. Available via http://www.legislation.gov.uk/ukpga/2001/15/pdfs/ukpga_20010015_en.pdf. Accessed 10 Jun 2017

Joint Formulary Committee (2008) British National Formulary. London: British Medical Association and Royal Pharmaceutical Society of Great Britain.7 Apr 2012

Medicinal Products Prescription by Nurses etc. Act (1992) Chapter 28. Available via http://www.legislation.gov.uk/ukpga/1992/28/introduction/enacted?view=plain. Accessed 10 Jun 2017

Medicines Act (1968) c.67. Available via http://www.legislation.gov.uk/ukpga/1968/67/contents. Accessed 10 Jun 2017

NICE and BNF (n.d.) Nurse Prescribers Formulary for Community Practitioners. Available via https://www.evidence.nhs.uk/formulary/bnfc/current/nurse-prescribers-formulary/nurse-prescribers-formulary-for-community-practitioners. Accessed 10 Jun 2017

Nursing and Midwifery Council (2006) Standards of Proficiency for Nurse and Midwife Prescribers. NMC, London

Nursing and Midwifery Council (2009) Standards of Proficiency for Nurse Prescribers without a Specialist Practice Qualification to Prescribe from the Community Practitioner Formulary. Available via https://www.nmc.org.uk/standards/additional-standards/standards-of-proficiency-for-nurse-and-midwife-prescribers/.

NICE (2016) A competency framework for all prescribers. Available via . https://www.rpharms.com/resources/frameworks/prescribers-competency-framework. Accessed 10 Jun 2017

The Medicines for Human Use (Prescribing) (Miscellaneous Amendments) Order (2006). Available via http://www.psni.org.uk/wp-content/uploads/2012/10/pharmacist-prescribing-pom-order.pdf. Accessed 10 Jun 2017

The Misuse of Drugs (Amendment No.2) (England, Wales and Scotland) Regulations (2012) 2012 No. 973. Available via https://www.gov.uk/government/news/nurse-and-pharmacist-independent-prescribing-changes-announced. Accessed 10 Jun 2017

The Pharmaceutical Society (2013) Standards and guidance for pharmacist prescribers. Available via http://www.psni.org.uk/wp-content/uploads/2012/09/Standards-and-Guidance-for-Pharmacist-Prescribing-April-2013.pdf. Accessed 10 Jun 2017

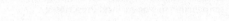

# Part I
# Non-medical Prescribing in Scotland, Wales and Northern Ireland

# Chapter 2
# Non-medical Prescribing in Scotland

**Andrew Rideout**

**Abstract**  Although prescribing was a nursing role in the earliest days of the profession, for over a hundred years nurses lost the legal right to prescribe. However, the last twenty years has seen the re-emergence of a diverse prescribing role, suited to the varied populations and clinical settings found across Scotland.

This chapter outlines the factors within society and coming from Scottish Government policy that had given impetus to the prescribing role in Scotland – possibly at a faster rate than the rest of the United Kingdom. There is also a discussion of both the growth in prescribing activity, and variations in prescribing activity across Scottish Health Boards, and a brief review of some of the literature about the wider prescribing context, including a number of case reports and studies that show the extent of prescribing across Scotland.

**Keywords**  Nurse • Nursing • Nurse practitioner • Advanced nurse practitioner • Advanced practitioner • Nurse prescriber • Nurse independent prescriber • Non-medical prescriber • Non-medical prescribing • Long-

A. Rideout
NHS Dumfries and Galloway, Dumfries, UK
e-mail: Andrew.rideout@nhs.net

© Springer International Publishing AG 2017

P.M. Franklin (ed.), *Non-medical Prescribing in the United Kingdom*,
DOI 10.1007/978-3-319-53324-7_2

17

term conditions • Long-term condition management •
Crown Report • *British National Formulary* • Scottish
Government • United Kingdom • Autonomy • Prescribing
Prescriptions • Acute care • Secondary care

The profession of nursing for lay people (principally women)
can be thought of as starting in 1833 when a nursing institute
started in Germany (Robinson 2005) and which later saw
Florence Nightingale as one of its students (Whyte 2010).
Around the same time, in Jamaica, Mary Seacole was following in her mother's trade as a healer, but honed her skills
in the frequent cholera epidemics and developed a more
scientific basis to her practice to become a nurse or "doc-
tress" (Robinson 2005) whose role included diagnosis, surgery and prescribing. Both of these early nursing pioneers
came to public attention for their nursing work in the
Crimea caring for soldiers. Whilst Florence Nightingale took
a leading role in public health and statistics, Mary Seacole
developed a wide clinical role and has been described as the
first nurse practitioner (Messmer and Parchment 1998). This
initial autonomous role for nurses was quickly brought into
a more subservient role in relation to medicine (Cutcliffe
and Wieck 2008; Hallett and Fealy 2009) and remained in
that position for over a 100 years, with the status quo being
maintained by both the medical and nursing professions
(Mitchell 2002; Esterhuizen 2006; Hallett and Fealy 2009).
However, there has been an increasing desire for greater
professional identity and autonomy in nursing (Watson
1999), and this has run alongside the development of new
(or redevelopment of old) nursing roles.
    A vision for a non-medical prescribing role within the United
Kingdom was officially laid out over 25 years ago with the publication of the *Crown Report* (*the Report of the Advisory Group on
Nurse Prescribing*) (DoH 1989) which identified patient and pro-

fessional benefits from this area of role expansion, including faster access to care for patients, better inter-professional communication and more appropriate use of staff and their skills. At this time the NHS across the United Kingdom operated as one unit, but since the devolution of much government activity to the newly established Scottish Government in 1999 Scotland has developed its own path for non-medical prescribing, as legislative changes have allowed.

In line with England, initially prescribing was limited to nurses with a community (health visitor or district nurse) qualification, from a very limited formulary. However, in 2006, both the range of professionals and the formulary were opened up to include all nurses or pharmacists with a further recordable prescribing qualification, who were now able to prescribe from most of the *British National Formulary* (BNF) for most conditions. Further changes in 2007 and 2012 to legislation and professional guidance have opened up non-medical prescribing to other allied health professionals and to include unlicensed and off-license drugs and the prescribing of controlled drugs with the same freedoms given to medically trained prescribers. There is some evidence that until the opening of the full formulary to non-medical prescribers in 2006, prescribing was a small part of nurses' workload, with only 25% of qualified prescribers issuing more than one prescription a year in 2006, increasing to 43% in 2010, by which point 72% of independent nurse prescribers were actively prescribing (Drennan et al. 2014).

Although non-medical prescribing is a devolved responsibility within Scotland, there was little delay in the implementation of prescribing, and in 2006 the Scottish Government (formerly the Scottish Executive) published *Non Medical Prescribing in Scotland: Guidance for Nurse Independent Prescribers and for Community Practitioner Nurse Prescribers in Scotland: A Guide for Implementation* (Scottish Executive 2006a) which both explained the legal basis for nurse prescribing and the Scottish Government's vision for it within the broader health service. The policy paper, *Delivering Care, Enabling Health: Harnessing the*

*Nursing, Midwifery and Allied Health Professions' Contribution to Implementing Delivering for Health in Scotland* (Scottish Executive 2006b), was published the same year and identified non-medical prescribing as a key area of growth in the development of nurses' roles in delivering the NHS Scotland agendas, stating that this area was firmly driven by better quality of care for patients. The government perceived that patients would have easier and more equal access to healthcare, and healthcare professionals would use their time more appropriately and work more flexibly as a team, as a result of this change. Further reports have again emphasised the role of nurse prescribing (Scottish Executive 2006c, d, 2007a). Many of the Scottish Government *HEAT* targets (Scottish Executive 2007b) are supported by changes in medicine management and prescribing practices, and the current *Shifting the Balance of Care* agenda continues to emphasise the role of non-medical prescribing (Scottish Government 2009a). Some of these policy documents (Scottish Executive 2007b) specifically mention the role of nurse prescribing away from the traditional community setting, although development of community capability continues to be a growing emphasis for the government (Scottish Government 2009a). With the increasing confidence of the government and the professions in non-medical prescribing, this role has been identified as one of the 20 key high impact changes within the NHS to change the way that care is delivered within Scotland (Scottish Government 2009b).

Similar developments have happened internationally during the same period (An Bord Altranais 2005; Kroezen et al. 2011), as the role of nurses has developed, and health delivery services have increasingly struggled to meet the demand upon them, both due to changes in the patient population and a shortage of medically qualified practitioners. The United Kingdom gives its non-medical prescribers the highest level of prescribing autonomy possible, with responsibilities and rights that are exactly equivalent to medical prescribers and are therefore greater than in some comparable countries (Kroezen et al. 2011).

Although there has been an increase of 17% (to almost 17,000) in the number of doctors in Scotland in the 10 years to 2014 (ISD 2007, 2014a, 2015), the effect of implementing the European Working Time Directive (DoH 2009) has reduced the number of doctors available 'on the shop floor' at any time. At the same time nurse and allied health professionals have been developing their roles and competencies (Scottish Executive 2006b) and moving into areas that were traditionally seen as a medical domain. The transfer of tasks between medicine and nursing has been ongoing for many years, but the process has accelerated over the last 20 years, with the first group of nurse practitioners graduating in the United Kingdom in 1991. Before this, informally trained nurse practitioners were already working, primarily in emergency departments, seeing around 3% of all patients (Read et al. 1992). Cooper et al. (2001) found that 10 years later, 40% of Scottish emergency departments had some level of nurse practitioner service, and the following year Horrocks et al. (2002) were able to conduct a systematic review of 34 papers examining the role of nurse practitioners in primary care, which concluded that nurse practitioners were well accepted by patients, with equivalent health outcomes and quality of care to doctors, although at a greater unit cost per patient.

Alongside changes in the workforce have been changes in the population requiring healthcare. These changes have led to increasing demands upon the NHS and can be considered to be caused by a combination of the increasing ageing population, persistent lifestyle factors that lead to a greater chronic disease burden within society (Lee et al. 2012) and greater expectations from the public.

These role developments have been supported at governmental level by the NHS Education for Scotland Advanced Practice Toolkit (NHS Education for Scotland 2008), which has been the Scottish Government's way of supporting previous policy documents such as *Framework for Developing Nursing Roles*

(Scottish Executive 2005) and *Modernising Nursing Careers* (Scottish Executive 2006c).

Whilst between 1999 and 2006 there was a 76% increase in the NHS Scotland budget (Scottish Executive 2006b), and although the NHS within Scotland was charged with making 2% year on year savings at the start of the decade (Scottish Government 2009b), following the Referendum the Scottish Government budget proposed a slight 'real terms' increase in NHS budget of 0.01% (Scottish Government 2014). However, this virtual financial budgetary standstill is to be achieved alongside service improvements (Scottish Government 2014), including:

- Increased patient contact
- Improved quality
- Reduced cost
- Greater levels of cash releasing efficiency for reinvestment in frontline patient care
- A more productive workplace culture
- Greater innovation in the use of technology to support efficiency
- Greater patient throughput particularly in high volume areas

The government states that one of the ways that these targets can be met is by the use of *toolkits to support demand, capacity, scheduling, skill mix management and rostering at a local level building on work done by NES and Nursing Directorate* (Scottish Government 2009b), which could be seen as encouraging the development of advanced nursing roles within the organisation. Prescribing is now seen as a key element to many advanced nursing roles across Scotland.

One of the continuous technological changes within healthcare is in the area of pharmaceuticals, and this represents a huge financial burden on the NHS (costing approximately £200 per person or £1.15bn in total per year (ISD 2014c) and for the first time in 2016 exceeds the staffing costs of some NHS organisations (Beardon 2016). For this reason a previous government stopped the implementation of nurse prescribing in 1992 from a fear that the costs would be unaffordable (Baird 2003), and although the number of prescription items prescribed by nurses grew from fewer than 2000 in 1996/1997 to over 880,000 by 2008/2009, and to just under 1.7 million items at a total cost of £20.6m in community settings alone by 2015/2016 (Paulley and Watson 2016), there is evidence that nurses prescribe more carefully and with greater cost awareness than doctors (Scottish Government 2009c).

As well as the increase in prescribing activity by non-medical prescribers already described (an 18% increasing in active prescribing between 2006 and 2010 (Drennan et al. 2014)), the number of prescribers continues to increase. In 2010 it was reported that there were 53,813 prescribers registered with the Nursing and Midwifery Council, of whom 19,137 (35.6%) were full independent prescribers (Culley 2010). By 2014 the number of non-medical prescribers had continued to increase to 65,364, but by this stage 29,226 (44.7%) of these prescribers were full independent prescribers (Blake 2014). However, within Scotland the proportion of independent prescribers is even greater, with 3052 (48.1%) out of a total of 6348 non-medical prescribers (Blake 2014). As there were 1985 clinical nurse specialists recorded in Scotland at the same time (ISD 2014b), this suggests that much of the non-medical prescribing work is undertaken by generalist nurses, albeit practising at an advanced level. When compared to England and Wales (Latter et al. 2011) where 2–3% of nurses are reported as being independent prescribers, a higher proportion of the Scottish workforce, at 5.2%, have this qualification.

Although there are case reports and discussions of nurse prescribing being practised in increasing numbers of acute care settings (Jones 2009), by 2006 only one in four prescribers was working in secondary care (Courtenay and Carey 2008), although almost half of prescribers undergoing training were based in secondary care (Bradley et al. 2005). Comparison of data from various sources (Culley 2010; Drennan et al. 2014) suggests that by 2010 between 30% and 32% of independent prescribers were based in secondary care. Recent unreleased figures (Beattie 2015) indicate that within Scotland this number may now be close to 60% of independent prescribers working in secondary care.

As with many earlier studies, a study within the north-west region of England by Hacking and Taylor (2010) also identified a majority (approximately two-thirds) of non-medical prescribers being placed within the primary care setting. A sizable minority (17%) were not prescribing at the time of the study, with about one in eight (14%) having never prescribed (Hacking and Taylor 2010). However, they report this percentage as being higher than previous studies, and the main reason given was organisational barriers rather than lack of confidence. Anecdotally the same situation is thought to exist within Scotland, with many of the early prescribers (community-based health visitors and district nurses) finding that they did not have the support or scope within their roles to develop their practice. However, newer services, developed since the expansion of non-medical prescribing, and incorporating prescribing as a core function have not had the same problem. The diversity of roles across Scotland has included sole clinical practitioners in remote and rural (or island based) community hospitals (Moss 2016); nurse evaluation and management of polypharmacy in the elderly in one remote and rural health board (Moss 2016); a non-medical (pharmacist)-led project to review and manage the pharmaceutical treatment of the frail elderly in a different remote and rural health board, leading to savings of £13k in the first 6 months (Kennedy et al. 2016); the development of a specialist children's palliative care service covering the whole of Scotland (Crooks et al. 2016); managing complex patients in police custody, many with dual diagnosis (drug/alcohol misuse and mental health problems) (Davidson 2015; Muirhead

2016); new interventions to improve the care of patients attending a specialist sexual health clinic in Scotland's largest city (Rooney and Caulfield 2016).

Much of the literature around non-medical prescribing relates to the period before the role was opened up to all nurses and practice settings. It therefore concentrates on the experiences and competencies of community nurses and the impact on patients and teams within the community and focuses on chronic disease management rather than acute interventions. However, the literature describing non-medical prescribing roles in acute care settings continues to grow and now encompasses advanced practice roles (Crathern et al. 2016; McDonnell et al. 2015), critical care and retrieval roles (Davies et al. 2016; Jackson and Carberry 2015; Topple et al. 2016), ward-based specialties (Hale et al. 2014; McDonnell et al. 2015) and acute outpatient and emergency department settings (Black 2012; Monitor 2014; Pearce and Winter 2014).

Although there are limited data, there is evidence of considerable variations that exist between Scottish Health Boards in prescribing patterns (SAPG 2011, Calderwood 2016), which are probably explained in part by human factors. A scoping study (Rideout 2015) of non-medical prescribing within acute care has demonstrated a broad range of prescribing, but also suggested unexplained differences existed in prescribing practices by nurses in similar roles with similar patient groups. This study also showed increased confidence in prescribing, with nurses prescribing from every section of the BNF, which compares to an earlier study (Drennan et al. 2014), which showed that there were groups of drugs which nurses were not prescribing at all. This concept of growing confidence in the prescribing role is supported by a study (Hacking and Taylor 2010) which found that 60% of non-medical prescribers issued more than ten prescriptions each week and 29% issued more than 20 prescriptions—the authors highlight this as being an increase in prescribing frequency compared to previous studies, suggesting that non-medical prescribers may be finding themselves increasingly comfortable in their role and finding greater usefulness in the role—indeed 57% of respondents thought that over half of their time was spent in prescribing-related activities. However, these authors did also find that non-medical prescribers were mainly (58%) prescribing in a limited (less than four) range of conditions in which they were highly knowledgeable, with only 5% of respondents prescribing as generalists (i.e. across a range of conditions and within a wide formulary). However, another recent Scottish study, specifically looking at prescribing patterns of generalist prescribers, found that in this group 100% of respondents prescribed on most days, with 79% prescribing several times on most days and 68% stating that they prescribed across a broad range of conditions (Rideout 2016).

Key to the successful implementation and development of non-medical prescribing in Scotland has been the close collaboration between the Scottish Government, Health Boards, NHS Education for Scotland (www.nes.scot.nhs.uk) and Higher Education Institutes. In practical terms the government has provided significant financial support to Health Boards to allow staff to undergo training, but additionally, representatives of the four groups have met four times a year to share best practice, develop and implement strategy, peer review prescribing practice and governance through visits across Scotland, and organise an annual national conference at no cost to attendees. This strong sense of working in partnership, longstanding supportive relationships, and the practical nature of the Prescribing Leads' Group has given the health service in Scotland a shared direction and forum for identifying and solving problems over the years.

In summary, non-medical prescribing has developed both nationally and internationally to meet a patient need and support development of services. There is some evidence that the non-medical prescribing role has been taken up to a greater extent in Scotland than the rest of the United Kingdom, and a greater proportion of Scottish prescribers work within acute and secondary care.

# References

An Bord Altranais (2005) Review of nurses and midwives in the prescribing and administration of medicinal products. An Bord Altranais, Dublin

Baird A (2003) Nurse prescribing—how did we get here? J Community Nurs 17(4):4

Beardon P (2016) Re: prescribing costs. In: Rideout A (ed). NHS Dumfries & Galloway, Dumfries

Beattie J (2015) Non medical prescriber numbers—September 2014—summary table. In: Rideout A (ed). Scottish Government, Edinburgh

Black A (2012) Non-medical prescribing by nurse practitioners in accident & emergency and sexual health: a comparative study. J Adv Nurs 69(3):535–545

Blake A (2014) Re: from website: new FOI request (email). In: Rideout A (ed). NMC, London

Bradley E, Campbell P, Nolan P (2005) Nurse prescribers: who are they and how do they perceive their role? J Adv Nurs 51(5):439–448

Calderwood C (2016) Realistic Medicine: Chief Medical Officer's Annual Report 2014-15. Scottish Government, Edinburgh

Cooper MA, Hair S, Ibbotson TR et al (2001) The extent and nature of emergency nurse practitioner services in Scotland. Accid Emerg Nurs 9(2):123–129

Courtenay M, Carey N (2008) Nurse independent prescribing and nurse supplementary prescribing practice: national survey. J Adv Nurs 61(3):291–299

Crathern L, Clark S, Evans D et al (2016) Developing an advanced neonatal nurse practitioner (ANNP) programme: a conversation on the process from both a service and education perspective. J Neonatal Nurs 22(1):2–8

Crooks H, Porter C, Cowling K et al (2016) Evaluation of non-medical prescribing in a children's hospice service. Scottish Government national non-medical prescribing conference, CHAS, Edinburgh

Culley F (2010) Professional considerations for nurse prescribers. Nurs Stand 24(43):55–60

Cutcliffe JR, Wieck KL (2008) Salvation or damnation: deconstructing nursing's aspirations to professional status. J Nurs Manag 16(5):499–507

Davidson J (2015) Nursing in police custody: creating a professional identity. Br J Nurs 24:1160–1161

Davies JK, Lynch F, Nyman A et al (2016) The role and scope of retrieval nurse practitioners in the UK. Nurs Crit Care 21(4):243–251

DoH (1989) Report of the advisory group on nurse prescribing (The Crown Report). Department of Health, London

DoH (2009) The European working time directive for trainee doctors—implementation update. Department of Health, London

Dowding D, Spilsbury K, Thompson C et al (2009) The decision making of heart failure specialist nurses in clinical practice. J Clin Nurs 18(9):1313–1324

Drennan VM, Grant R, Harris R (2014) Trends over time in prescribing by English primary care nurses: a secondary analysis of a national prescription database. BMC Health Serv Res 14:54

Eccles M, Grimshaw J, Johnston M et al (2007) Applying psychological theories to evidence-based clinical practice: identifying factors predictive of managing upper respiratory tract infections without antibiotics. Implement Sci 2:26

Esterhuizen P (2006) Is the professional code still the cornerstone of clinical nursing practice? J Adv Nurs 53(1):104–110

Hacking S, Taylor J (2010) An evaluation of the scope and practice of non medical prescribing in the North West for NHS North West (Final Report). University of Central Lancashire, Preston

Hale A, Martin J, Coombes ID et al (2014) A pilot study to assess the appropriateness of prescribing from a collaborative pharmacist prescribing study in a surgical pre admission clinic. J Pharma Care Health Sys 1(3). doi:10.4172/2376-0419.1000110

Hall J, Noyce P, Cantrill J (2008) Why do district nurse prescribers alter their prescribing patterns? Br J Community Nurs 13(11):507–513

Hallett C, Fealy GM (2009) Guest editorial: nursing history and the articulation of power. J Clin Nurs 18(19):2681–2683

Hay A, Bradley E, Nolan P (2004) Supplementary nurse prescribing. Nurs Stand 18(41):33–39

Horrocks S, Anderson E, Salisbury C (2002) Systematic review of whether nurse practitioners working in primary care can provide equivalent care to doctors. BMJ 324(7341):819–823

ISD (2007) HCHS medical and dental staff by time, speciality. NHS Board and Region. http://www.isdscotland.org/Health-Topics/Workforce/Historic-Data/index.asp - 1. Accessed 18 Dec 2016

ISD (2014a) Medical & dental staff in post. http://www.isdscotland.org/Health-Topics/Workforce/Medical-and-Dental/. Accessed 18 Dec 2016

ISD (2014b) Nursing and midwifery workforce. Available via http://www.isdscotland.org/Health-Topics/Workforce/Nursing-and-Midwifery/. Accessed 11 June 2017

ISD (2014c) Prescribing & medicines: prescription cost analysis financial year 2013/14. NHS National Services, Scotland, Edinburgh

ISD (2015) Number (headcount) of GPs in post, by gender & age group, 2004 to 2014—Scotland. Available at http://www.isdscotland.org/Health-Topics/General-Practice/Workforce-and-Practice-Populations/Workforce. Accessed 18 Dec 2016

Jackson A, Carberry M (2015) The advance nurse practitioner in critical care: a workload evaluation. Nurs Crit Care 20(2):71–77

Jones K (2009) Developing a prescribing role for acute care nurses. Nurs Manag 16(7):24–28

Kennedy E, Luoughran G, Dillett J (2016) Optimise: a novel approach to improving medicines management in frail, older adults. Paper presented at Scottish Government national non-medical prescribing conference, Queen Margaret University, Edinburgh, 25 May 2016

Kroezen M, van Dijk L, Groenewegen P et al (2011) Nurse prescribing of medicines in Western European and Anglo-Saxon countries: a systematic review of the literature. BMC Health Serv Res 11:127

Latter S, Blenkinsopp A, Smith A et al (2011) Evaluation of nurse and pharmacist independent prescribing. Department of Health, London

Lee IM, Shiroma EJ, Lobelo F et al (2012) Effect of physical inactivity on major non-communicable diseases worldwide: an analysis of burden of disease and life expectancy. Lancet 380(9838):219–229

McDonnell A, Goodwin E, Kennedy F et al (2015) An evaluation of the implementation of advanced nurse practitioner (ANP) roles in an acute hospital setting. J Adv Nurs 71(4):789–799

Messmer PR, Parchment Y (1998) Mary Grant Seacole: the first nurse practitioner. Clin Excell Nurse Pract 2(1):47–51

Mitchell T (2002) Becoming a nurse. Ashgate Publishing Ltd, Aldershot

Monitor (2014) Walk-in centre review: final report and recommendations. Monitor, London

Moss D (2016) Patient centred medication in primary care. Paper presented at Scottish Government national non-medical prescribing conference, Queen Margaret University, Edinburgh, 25 May 2016

Muirhead B (2016) Evidence based prescribing? An audit from a nurse led custody healthcare service. Paper presented at Scottish Government national non-medical prescribing conference, Queen Margaret University, Edinburgh, 25 May 2016

NHS Education for Scotland (2008) Advanced practice toolkit. Available at http://www.advancedpractice.scot.nhs.uk/. Accessed 18 Dec 2016

O'Malley P (2007) Order no harm: evidence-based methods to reduce prescribing errors for the clinical nurse specialist. Clin Nurse Spec 21(2):68–70

Otway C (2001) Informal peer support: a key to success for nurse prescribers. Br J Community Nurs 6(11):586

Paulley G, Watson H (2016) Non-medical prescribing: information request IR2016–02440 (Personal Correspondence). Information Services Division, NHS Scotland, Glasgow

Pearce C, Winter H (2014) Review of non-medical prescribing among acute and community staff. Nurs Manag 20(10):22–26

Read SM, Jones NM, Williams BT (1992) Nurse practitioners in accident and emergency departments: what do they do? BMJ 305(6867): 1466–1470

Rideout A (2015) Measuring non-medical prescribing. Paper presented at Faculty of Public Health Scottish Conference, Peebles, 5th November 2015

Rideout A (2016) Nurse prescribing in out of hours. Paper presented at non-medical prescribing in paediatrics and child health conference, Hallam Conference Centre, London, 5 October 2016

Robinson J (2005) Mary Seacole. Constable and Robinson, London

Rooney E, Caulfield P (2016) Proposal to explore the impact of non-medical prescribers in management of post-exposure prophylaxis against HIV. Paper presented at Scottish Government national non-medical prescribing conference, Queen Margaret University, Edinburgh, 26 May 2016

Ryan-Woolley B, McHugh G, Luker KA (2007) Prescribing by specialist nurses in cancer and palliative care: results of a national survey. Palliat Med 21(4):273–277

SAPG (2011) Primary care prescribing indicators: annual report 2010–11. ISD Scotland, Edinburgh

Scottish Executive (2005) Framework for developing nursing roles. Scottish Executive Health Department, Edinburgh

Scottish Executive (2006a) Non medical prescribing in Scotland: guidance for nurse independent prescribers and for community practitioner nurse prescribers in Scotland: a guide for implementation. Scottish Executive Health Department, Edinburgh

Scottish Executive (2006b) Delivering care, enabling health: harnessing the nursing, midwifery and allied health professions' contribution to implementing delivering for health in Scotland. Scottish Executive Health Department, Edinburgh

Scottish Executive (2006c) Modernising nursing careers: setting the direction. Scottish Executive Health Department, Edinburgh

Scottish Executive (2006d) Non-medical prescribing in Scotland. Scottish Executive Health Department, Edinburgh

Scottish Executive (2007a) Co-ordinated, integrated and fit for purpose: a delivery framework for adult rehabilitation in Scotland. Scottish Executive Health Department, Edinburgh

Scottish Executive (2007b) Better health, better care: action plan. Scottish Executive Health Department, Edinburgh

Scottish Government (2009a) Improving outcomes by shifting the balance of care: delivery framework. Scottish Government, Edinburgh

Scottish Government (2009b) NHS Scotland efficiency and productivity programme: delivery framework. Available via http://www.gov.scot/Publications/2009/06/22125603/0. Accessed 11 June 2017

Scottish Government (2009c) A safe prescription. Scottish Government, Edinburgh

Scottish Government (2014) Scottish budget: draft budget 2015–16. Scottish Government, Edinburgh

Stenner K, Courtenay M (2008) The role of inter-professional relationships and support for nurse prescribing in acute and chronic pain. J Adv Nurs 63(3):276–283

Topple M, Ryan B, McKay R et al (2016) Features of an intensive care based medical emergency team nurse training program in a University Teaching Hospital. Aust Crit Care 29(1):46–49

Watson J (1999) Postmodern nursing and beyond. Churchill Livingstone, Edinburgh

Whyte A (2010) Relighting the lamp. Nurs Stand 24(18):18–20

# Chapter 3
# Non-medical Prescribing in Wales: Implementation and Governance

**Eleri Mills**

**Abstract**  There have been changes made to the United Kingdom (UK) wide medicines legislation-permitting non-medical prescribing in the UK. Consequently as a result of this, it is up to each devolved administration to decide how it is implemented within its National Health Service. In order to enable this to happen, changes to NHS Wales Regulations have been made. In Wales along with the other three countries in the UK, the last two and a half decades has seen significant developments in non-medical prescribing policy and practice, with other healthcare professionals gaining prescribing rights. This has resulted due to the extension of prescribing authority, to nurse and midwives initially, and since, to pharmacists and certain allied health professions. Indeed, this has been an exciting development for the healthcare profession in Wales, which has had to respond to significant changes in how patient care and health provision are delivered.

E. Mills
School of Social and Life Sciences, Wrexham Glyndŵr University,
Mold Road, Wrexham, Wales LL11 2AW, UK
e-mail: e.mills@glyndwr.ac.uk

© Springer International Publishing AG 2017
P.M. Franklin (ed.), *Non-medical Prescribing in the United Kingdom*,
DOI 10.1007/978-3-319-53324-7_3

**Keywords**  Cumberlege Report • Wales • Prescribing of
medicines • Supply of medicines, and Administration of
medicines • District nurses • Health visitors • Devolved
country • Community nurses • Pharmacists • Repeat
prescribing • Multi-professional training • Prescription
only medicines order • Nurse • Community nurse •
Physiotherapist • Podiatrist • Radiographer • Dietician •
Optometrist • Audit • Monitoring • Clinical governance •
Continuing professional development

## 3.1  Implementation of Non-medical Prescribing: Nurse Prescribing Formulary

As is well published, nurse prescribing was originally recommended in the Cumberlege Report back in 1986 (DoH 1986). The Report of the Review of Prescribing, Supply and Administration of Medicines (Department of Health 1989) advised ministers in the UK on how introducing nurse prescribing could improve the patient care given to patients within the community. Dr. June Crown chaired this group, and thus the report became known nationally as the First Crown Report. Ten years later, the final report on the Review of Prescribing, Supply and Administration (DoH 1999) recommended that:

> *The legal authority to prescribe should be extended to include new professional groups and*
> *Introduced the concept of an Independent Prescriber and a Dependent Prescriber. The term Dependent Prescriber was later changed to Supplementary Prescriber.*

Within Wales the first cohort of District Nurses and Health Visitors qualified as prescribers towards the end of 2000, with further cohorts completing the educational preparation at approved Academic Educational Institutions thereafter.

## 3.2 Implementation of Supplementary Prescribing: Wales Context

As a devolved country, the situation in Wales relied heavily on Welsh policies in order to drive non-medical prescribing forward, and subsequently many policies were published in response to this. There is no doubt that the development of non-medical prescribing in Wales is a dynamic process, and this is reflected in the number of policies published. In 2001, Improving Health in Wales—A Plan for the NHS with its Partners (NAW 2001a) was published and stated that the implementation of the Review of Prescribing, Supply and Administration of Medicines by 2004 should provide patients with more convenient and efficient access to medicines and increase the number of professionals who can write prescriptions and take on the responsibility for their administration and effectiveness. Consequently, a Report of the Task and Finish Group on Prescribing was established in 2001 to consider options to improve the prescribing of drugs (NAW 2001b). Interestingly, the report made almost 100 recommendations and was presented to the Health and Social Services Committee in March 2001. Some of the key recommendations were identified from this report by the task and finish group (NAW 2001b) that was established by the minister for Health and Social Services to consider the options to improve the prescribing of drugs and included the following:

- There is a need for a more efficient, safe and more streamlined system of repeat prescribing that is easy for the patient to use.
- All staff undertaking prescribing should be appropriately trained and undertake accreditation to carry out these functions, within the recognised limits of competence.
- All prescribers should be given training in communication and counselling.

- The role of pharmacists and nurses as supplementary prescribers must be developed so as to offer patients regular dialogue about, and monitoring of, their medicines.
- There should be a continuing drive for more effective prescribing (NAW 2001b).

Within 3 months in July 2001, *Improving Health in Wales—The Future of Primary Care* was published by the National Assembly for Wales (NAW 2001c). This document focused on supporting the legal authority to prescribe for other professionals. Three main themes emerged. Firstly, assurance had to be given to nurses working in primary care that they could have access to an accredited educational programme, which had to include an appropriate prescribing module. Secondly, it acknowledged the role that nurses and health visitors who work in the community had in improving access for patients through nurse prescribing initiatives. Thirdly, it made reference to the role that pharmacists had in prescribing within repeat prescribing.

In May 2002, *MLX 284 proposals for supplementary prescribing by nurses and pharmacists and proposed amendments to the prescription only medicines (human use) order 1997* was circulated (MCA 2002). Following the evaluation of the responses, the Welsh Health and Social Services minister announced intention to support the introduction of supplementary prescribing in Wales. This was different to that in England where nurses were undertaking both independent and supplementary prescribing programmes. Thereafter, in September 2002 the Welsh Assembly Government published a consultation document *Remedies for Success—A Strategy for Pharmacy in Wales* (WAG 2002). The main theme within this document was a strategy for pharmacy in Wales, stating that the Welsh Assembly government was also committed to the extension of supplementary prescribing rights to pharmacists by 2004. A task and finish group was established in August 2003 to drive supplementary prescribing. Funding was granted by the Health and Social Services Minister in a plenary session to Assembly Members on 20 November 2003, that £0.5M would be made available to educate and train around 250 nurses and pharmacists to become the first supplementary prescribers to qualify in Wales in 2004.

The All Wales Medicines Strategy Group (AWMSG) was given responsibility to implement the recommendations of the task and finish group on prescribing in Wales and established a task and finish group to take forward the development of supplementary prescribing by nurses and pharmacists in Wales (Mitchell 2003). The task and finish group project scope was to develop a training programme accredited by the appropriate professional bodies for training nurses and pharmacists to become supplementary prescribers. As part of this, consideration was given to the variety of delivery methods available and multi-professional training packages. The group also considered whether there was a need for a Wales-specific syllabus or whether there was a programme already being delivered that may be used in Wales. Delivery of the programme was considered as to whether there was a need for separate programme for nurses and pharmacists; a multi-professional programme with nurses and pharmacists attending a common core programme with separate elements based on the differences in background experience and knowledge; an all Wales programme provided by a single centre or multiple centres across Wales; and separate programmes developed by each Academic Educational Institution with consideration given to distance learning and computer packages (Mitchell 2003). Academic Educational Institutions were contacted to develop training programmes for supplementary prescribing by nurses and pharmacists and to provide training needs for the medical practitioners whose role was to provide the training and support in the practical element of the programme. Healthcare organisations were contacted about their commitment to the nurses' and pharmacists' supplementary prescribing programme, and they identified nurses and pharmacists to be trained based on service needs and independent doctor prescribers as medical practitioners who would provide the 12-day learning in practice element. Assistance was given with the allocation of training places to ensure equity and course viability and release funding as appropriate. Feedback was sought from students on the training programme to ensure standards were maintained and any difficulties addressed for future programmes. Procedures were developed to annotate professional registers and prescription pads made available to enable supplementary prescribers to prescribe with minimal delay following successful completion of the training programme (Mitchell 2003).

Possible constraints were identified, such as a non-recurring budget, the ability of the Academic Educational Institution to respond within the timeframe, and requirements of the Nursing and Midwifery Council for nurses and Royal Pharmaceutical Society of Great Britain for pharmacists' accreditation by Health Professions Wales. Difficulties in releasing pharmacists and nurses to undertake the training programme and difficulties associated with the medical practitioner providing the 12-day learning in practice were also identified (Mitchell 2003). It was decided that each of the universities would deliver the supplementary prescribing programme for nurses and pharmacists based on the guidance given by the task and finish group for supplementary prescribing and the approved professional bodies—Nursing and Midwifery Council (NMC) and the then Royal Pharmaceutical Society of Great Britain (RPSGB) in this case.

## 3.3  Implementation of Independent Prescribing: Wales Context

With the Department of Health (2004) policy document implying that nurses' skills and experiences should be developed to provide high-quality care, the Welsh approach was steered by the *Review of Health and Social Care in Wales* (Wanless 2003), and *Designed for Life: Creating World Class Health and Social Care for Wales* (WAG 2005). Between February and May 2005, a joint consultation between the Department of Health and the Medicines and Healthcare Products Regulatory Agency examined the options for the future of independent nurse prescribing. At the same time there was a similar consultation examining options for the introduction of independent prescribing by pharmacists. As was stated in the Crown report (DoH 1989), it was about providing benefits to patients by allowing greater access and faster and more accessible services.

The Committee on Safety of Medicines in November 2005 considered the responses from both consultations, and recommendations were made to Ministers that suitably qualified nurses and pharmacists should be able to prescribe licensed medicines, including some controlled drugs for nurses only, for any medical condition within their own competence. UK Ministers agreed with this proposal, and recommendations were announced on 10 November 2005. Consequently, the *Medicines for Human Use (Prescribing) (Miscellaneous Amendments) Order 2006 and associated medicines regulations* enabled nurses who train and qualify as 'nurse independent prescribers' to prescribe licensed medicines, including some controlled drugs for any medical condition within their own competence (HMSO 2006). In the case of pharmacists, there were some differences. Pharmacist independent prescribers at this time were not allowed to prescribe any controlled drug but allowed to prescribe licensed medicines within their own competence. The above amendments applied across the UK.

In 2006, the Department of Health published a guide to implementing nurse and pharmacist independent prescribing within the NHS in England; however, this was not enforced in Wales (DoH 2006). This was to increase patient choice, improve access to advice and services without compromising patient safety, appropriate use of skilled healthcare workforce, contribute to the introduction of more flexible working across the NHS and increase capacity to meet demand of new ways of working. By 2007 legislative changes were in place for Academic Educational Institutions to accredit programmes with students undergoing training to enable registration with the NMC and RPSGB as the professional regulatory body within a clinical governance framework.

Designed for life, Creating World Class Health and Social Care for Wales in the twenty-first century (WAG 2005) was the policy driver behind the implementation of independent prescribing in Wales, by extending prescribing responsibilities to non-medical professions. The rationale for supplementary prescribing to also include independent prescribing in Wales was as a result of increased patient choice, improved access to advice and services without compromising patient safety, appropriate use of skilled healthcare workforce and contribution to the introduction of more flexible team working across the NHS with increased capacity to meet demand of new ways of working.

Changes to the Prescription Only Medicines Order were passed on 1 May 2006, which was UK wide. Changes to NHS regulations were for devolved administrators who were from Wales only, and it was expected to come into force in December 2006. Once agreed, it was progressed through the Primary Care Division of the Welsh Assembly Government. The task and finish group for independent prescribing reported to the All Wales Medicines Strategy Group with a first meeting on 7 April 2006 where a Chair was appointed and subgroups established. It was envisaged that the independent prescribing programme would be a multidisciplinary programme with all five Academic Educational Institutions in Wales currently delivering the supplementary prescribing programme seeking approval to deliver the independent prescribing programme from the respective professional bodies.

Due to the devolved government in Wales, changes to *National Health Service (Miscellaneous Amendments concern-*

*ing independent nurse prescribers, supplementary prescribers, nurse independent prescribers and pharmacist independent prescribers) (Wales) Regulations 2007 (SI 2007/205 (W.19)* came into effect in Wales on 1 February 2007 (National Assembly for Wales 2007). In February 2007, *NHS regulations (Wales) (SI 2007/205 (W.19)* were also amended to allow registered chiropodists and podiatrists; physiotherapists; radiographers, diagnostic or therapeutic; and optometrists to practise as supplementary prescribers once qualified (National Assembly for Wales 2007).

The *National Health Service (Miscellaneous amendments concerning independent nurse prescribers, supplementary prescribers, nurse independent prescribers and pharmacist independent prescriber) (Wales) Regulations 2007 (SI 2007/205 (W.19)* (National Assembly for Wales 2007) set out the definition of supplementary prescriber, nurse independent prescriber and pharmacist independent prescriber. The definitions were amended in July 2010 in respect of *Wales by The National Health Service (Miscellaneous Amendments relating to Independent Prescribing) (Wales) Regulation 2010* (Welsh Statutory Instruments 2010). This latest change clarifies that the term 'independent nurse prescriber' refers to those nurses and midwives approved by the Nursing and Midwifery Council able to prescribe drugs, medicines and appliances as a 'community practitioner nurse prescriber'.

On 23 April 2012, the *Misuse of Drugs (Amendment No 2) (England, Wales and Scotland) Regulations 2012* came into force (HMSO 2012) and amended the *Misuse of Drugs 2001 for England, Scotland and Wales* (HMSO 2001). As a consequence, nurse independent prescribers and pharmacist independent prescribers in Wales can prescribe a controlled drug within their level of competence, removing the previous limitations. The controlled drugs that can be prescribed are set out on schedules 2–5 of the *Misuse of Drugs Regulations 2001*. The changes do not apply to the prescribing of cocaine, diamorphine or dipipanone for the treatment of addiction (*Regulation 6B of the Misuse of Drugs Regulations 2001*) (HMSO 2001).

Nurses other than community practitioner nurse prescribers were initially allowed for supplementary prescribing rights only; however, at time of writing, nurses, physiotherapists, podiatrists, pharmacists and therapeutic radiographers have independent prescribing rights. In line with the rest of the UK, dieticians have been given supplementary prescribing rights. All five universities in Wales provide multi-professional non-medical prescribing education programmes. Currently the following educational programmes are available: supplementary prescribing for chiropodists and podiatrists and integrated independent and supplementary programme for nurses, pharmacists, chiropodist, podiatrists and physiotherapists. Independent and supplementary prescribing optometrists attend university courses in England or Scotland approved by the General Optical Council and are examined by the College of Optometrists. It is anticipated that independent prescribing courses will be available through Wales Optometry Postgraduate Education Centre in 2016 (WG 2015). Recent changes to legislation in the UK enable dieticians to undertake training as supplementary prescribers and therapeutic radiographers as independent and supplementary prescribers (HCPC 2016); however, medicine legislation has not been amended in Wales to date.

In Wales it is mandatory for all non-medical prescribers to successfully demonstrate their numeracy skills as part of their preparation for the role as prescriber. If this is not the case, a formal assessment will be required before they are permitted to practise in Wales. Optometrists are not required to undertake a numeracy test (WG 2015).

In Wales, each non-medical prescriber needs a doctor who will act as their designated supervising medical practitioner (DSMP). They provide supervision, support and opportunities to develop competence in prescribing and are involved in assessing that the independent/supplementary prescriber is competent. The DSMP role is the same as a designated medical prescriber (DMP) role in England. In line with the other three countries, currently there is no financial support given to DSMPs to support the independent/supplementary prescriber whilst shadowing clinical practice with their DSMP on the programme in Wales.

## 3.4 Audit and Monitoring of Prescribing Data in Wales

NHS Wales Informatics Service—Prescribing Services reimburses costs for dispensing contractors and provides essential prescribing information electronically to authorised users in Wales. Feedback on prescribing practice and trends are obtained via this system, which is particularly important for monitoring prescribing activity. All Local Health Boards in Wales have access to prescribing data using *Comparative Analysis System for Prescribing Audit* (*CASPA*) software systems and can access and provide information on medical and non-medical prescribing. General practices can have access to *CASPA* software for their individual practice and are required to register with NHS Wales Informatics Service—Prescribing Services to do so (WG 2015).

Any non-medical prescriber requiring NHSWP10 prescriptions, which are used in primary care and outpatient departments, must register with NHS Wales Informatics Service—Prescribing Services. Notification of the required details to National Health Service (NHS) Wales Informatics Service—Prescribing Services enables the setting up of automatic monitoring processes as well as allowing the provision of prescriber details to the print management supplier for the printing of personalised prescription pads. NHS Wales Informatics Service—Prescribing Services will register the non-medical prescriber against a Local Health Board (LHB) identified prescribing budget. If the non-medical prescriber is working at more than one location, for example, working at three general practices, a separate registration is required for each location. Prior to this the non-medical prescriber must ensure that they have discussed with the LHB in which area they intend to prescribe and their intention to prescribe prior to registering with NHS Wales Informatics Service—Prescribing Services. The appropriate person at the LHB must also sign the form before returning it to NHS Wales Informatics Service—Prescribing Services. Any change in prescriber circumstances must be reported to NHS Wales Informatics Service—Prescribing Services by the employer as soon as possible. The prescribing costs arising from WP10 prescriptions will be charged to the appropriate LHB prescribing budget. Within secondary care a non-medical prescriber whose prescriptions will be dispensed in the hospital should prescribe on standard hospital stationary using the All Wales Prescription Charts for inpatients, discharge prescription or outpatient prescription. Single sheet prescriptions are available to use with GP computer-generated systems, and the independent/supplementary prescriber should request the single sheet version of the WP10 as opposed to a pad from NHS Wales Informatics Service—Prescribing Services (WG 2015).

Within the NHS service provision in Wales, there have to be some workforce plans drawn up and LHBs producing a system of evaluation and planning to match prescribing needs. As stated in the latest edition of the *Non-medical Prescribing in Wales Guidance Document* (WG 2015), particular attention should be made to the needs of the population and how general practice services and dental prescribing services can be supported by non-medical prescribing. Within the document it suggests that with the LHB/Trust a network between nursing, pharmacy and medical leads is set up to develop an overall LHB/Trust non-medical strategy. It is very clear that the Welsh government is keen for opportunities to improve NHS service provision through the implementation of non-medical prescribing and that

LHBs/Trusts should aim to implement the use of non-medical prescribers. This information is clearly articulated in the *Non-medical Prescribing in Wales Guidance Document* (WG 2015), which is a useful document for all employers in Wales to refer to in respect of aspects of non-medical prescribing.

## 3.5  Clinical Governance: Continuing Professional Development

Education providers are responsible for maintaining the continuing professional development (CPD) needs of DSMPs in preparing their clinical and assessor skills for this role. All non-medical prescribers are required to maintain their currency with evidence and best practice in the management of conditions for which they prescribe including the use of the relevant medicines. The employer is also responsible for ensuring that the non-medical prescriber has access to relevant education and training provision. There is no doubt that appropriate CPD is a professional obligation for all NMPs. CPD is an integral part of the clinical governance process, alongside ensuring clear lines of responsibility and accountability for overall quality of clinical care; development of identified quality improvement programmes, including clinical audit; supporting evidence-based practice; implementation of clinical standards; monitoring of clinical care; workforce planning and development; and identification and effective management of risk. In Wales there is a range of methods of attaining CPD from various sources. All Wales Therapeutics and Toxicology Centre (AWTTC) delivers services in the fields of therapeutics and toxicology by bringing together, under one banner, five different NHS organisations that provide continuing support and advice relating to safe, clinically and cost-effective use of medicines in Wales. Resources include Patient Access to Medicine Service (PAMS) focusing on improving access to medicines. The Welsh Analytical Prescribing Support Unit (WAPSU) has published resources that have been endorsed by the All Wales Medicines Strategy Group. Their remit includes:

- *Analysing and reporting on medicines usage data*
- *Forecasting prescribing activity*
- *Developing guidelines and educational resources*
- *Facilitating the Wales Patient Access Scheme process*

There is also a link to the Welsh Medicines Resource Centre (WeMeRec). WeMeRec is a Welsh Education Resource Centre and is a source of independent information for all healthcare professionals and advisors working in Wales. They provide education in therapeutics, prescribing and behavioural change through a combination of digital and face-to-face learning opportunities. This is an organisation in Wales providing educational resources to multidisciplinary professionals to influence safe and effective prescribing. They provide multidisciplinary prescribing workshops and case studies and host an email discussion forum for non-medical prescribers. This can also be accessed via WeMeRec—www.wemerec.org. There is also a link to the Welsh National Poisons Unit (WNPU) and the Yellow Card Centre Wales (YCC Wales). The All Wales Medicines Strategy Group (AWMSG) also provides advice to the Minister for Health and Social Services in an effective, efficient and transparent manner on strategic medicines management and prescribing. There are key links to various documents that are applicable to all prescribers such as *Prescribing Dilemmas—A Guide for Prescribers* (AWMSG 2015).

Following successful completion of a non-medical prescribing programme, it is recommended that non-medical prescribers use the competency framework produced by the Royal Pharmaceutical Society (RPS 2016) to help inform their CPD needs, taking into account their profession and area of prescribing practice.

In line with other countries in the UK, the CPD needs of NMPs should be identified as part of their professional development plan and should be linked to the staff development/*Knowledge and Skills Framework* (KSF) process (DoH 2004). The NMP should be able to demonstrate evidence of continued competence. This could be done by the use of a professional portfolio, identifying any new medications and the conditions for which they have been prescribing, outside the normal sphere of practice. Evidence of ongoing CPD is forwarded to the NMP lead on a yearly basis, to be annotated on the local non-medical prescribing database. A personal prescribing formulary, signed by the appropriate supervising medical practitioner, is also considered by the NMP and the line manager to support prescribing in practice. The personal formulary is amended to show changes in prescribing practice during the year. NMPs are encouraged to identify their individual training needs with their line manager, and these should be included in their personal development plan. It is the responsibility of the NMP to ensure they remain up to date on therapeutics in the field of their prescribing practice and on changes in national and local prescribing policy. It is envisaged that all NMPs maintain their own knowledge through literature, professional networks such as the Association for Prescribing and clinical supervision to name a few. The recent updated published competency framework for all prescribers (RPS 2016) can also be used effectively to demonstrate competency and identify new areas for further development and updating by the non-medical prescriber from any profession. NMPs are also encouraged to develop networks with other non-medical prescribers who are prescribing within the same specialty or area of practice for peer support and supervision.

## 3.6   Summary

Since the publication of the Wanless Report in Wales (WAG 2005), there has been public recognition for the need to focus on the current government policy to improve health, reduce inequalities and promote social justice by improving access to healthcare services (WAG 2009). There is no doubt that the implementation of non-medical prescribing in Wales will contribute to the delivery of a high-quality, patient-centred service that will require flexibility in its role to achieve the aims of the NHS modernisation agenda.

It is evident that the Welsh Government has made a strong commitment to implementing non-medical prescribing within Wales. This is evident in the original Welsh Assembly policy drivers and their ambition for non-medical prescribing to evolve across the professions and become integrated in service delivery to improve patient care and access to medicines, by making their single encounter with the NHS more productive and efficient. We have also seen commitment to the concept of introducing non-medical prescribing in Wales in:

- Increased patient choice in accessing medicines
- Improved access to advice and services
- Appropriate use of skilled healthcare workforce
- Contribution to the introduction of more flexible team working across the NHS
- Increased capacity to meet demand of new ways of working
- Improvement in patient care without compromising patient safety (WG 2015)

Interestingly the Designed for Life (WAG 2005) policy document continues to support the modernisation agenda described within the 5-year Service, Workforce and Financial Framework (2010–2015) (WAG 2010). Together for Health—A 5-Year Vision of the NHS in Wales also refers to the vision for the NHS in 2016 supporting the ambition of a world-class health and social services in Wales (WG 2011). It is evident that the Welsh Government is supportive of non-medical prescribing and will continue to develop policies which will enable its expansion with Local Health Boards and Trusts in Wales to further implement the use of non-medical prescribers in the delivery of NHS provision within Wales (WG 2015).

The current prescribing rights for the non-medical professions are again evidence that the legal framework has been developed and established and is still evolving recognising that non-medical prescribing is essential in meeting the needs of the twenty-first-century healthcare provision.

It is clear that independent and supplementary prescribing is here to stay in Wales, and there is a need for further research to underpin the evidence base to support future developments. Certainly prescribing is a highly skilled activity that is high risk and therefore requires a skilled, safe and up-to-date prescribing practitioner working within healthcare services.

# References

All Wales Medicines Strategy Group (2015) Prescribing dilemmas—a guide for prescribers. All Wales Medicines Strategy Group, Cardiff

Department of Health (1989) Report of the advisory group on nurse prescribing (Crown Report). Department of Health, London

Department of Health (1999) Review of prescribing, supply and administration of medicines (Crown Final Report). Department of Health, London

Department of Health (2004) The NHS knowledge and skills framework and the development review process. Department of Health, London

Department of Health (2006) Improving patients' access to medicines: a guide to implementing nurse and pharmacist independent prescribing within the NHS in England. Department of Health, London

Department of Health and Social Security (1986) Neighbourhood nursing: a focus for care (Cumberlege Report). HMSO, London

HCPC (2016) Prescribing. Available via http://www.hcpc-uk.co.uk/aboutregistration/medicinesandprescribing/. Accessed 11 Jun 2017

HMSO (2001) Misuse of drugs regulations 2001 relating to nurse and pharmacist independent prescribing of controlled drugs (misuse of drugs (Amendment No.2) (England, Wales and Scotland) regulations 2012) (Statutory Instrument 2012/973). The Stationery Office, London

HMSO (2006) Statutory instruments 2006 No 915 the medicines for human use (prescribing) (miscellaneous amendments) order 2006. The Stationery Office, London

HMSO (2012) The misuse of drugs regulations 2012 relating to nurse and pharmacist independent prescribing of controlled drugs (Amendment

No.2) (England, Wales and Scotland) regulations 2012 No. 973. The
Stationery Office, London. Available via https://www.gov.uk/government/
news/nurse-and-pharmacist-independent-prescribing-changes-
announced. Accessed 11 Jun 2017

Medicines Control Agency (MCA) (2002) Proposals for supplementary
prescribing by nurses and pharmacists and proposed amendments to the
prescription only medicines (human use) order 1997. MLX 284.
Medicines Control Agency, London

Mitchell M (2003) Project initiation document—project to enable nurses and
pharmacists in Wales to become supplementary prescribers by developing and introducing an appropriate training programme. Unpublished

National Assembly for Wales (2001a) Improving health in Wales. A plan
for the NHS with its Partners. National Assembly for Wales, Cardiff

National Assembly for Wales (2001b) Report of the task and finish group
for prescribing in Wales. National Assembly for Wales, Cardiff

National Assembly for Wales (2001c) Improving health in Wales—the
future of primary care, Cardiff. National Assembly for Wales, Cardiff

National Assembly for Wales (2007) The National Health Service, (miscellaneous amendments concerning independent nurse prescribers, supplementary prescribers, nurse independent prescribers and pharmacist
independent prescribers) (Wales) regulations 2007. Statutory
Instruments 2007, No 205 (W.19). http://www.legislation.gov.uk/
changes/affected/wsi/2007. Accessed 17 Nov 2016

Royal Pharmaceutical Society (2016) A competency framework for all prescribers. Royal Pharmaceutical Society, Available via https://www.
rpharms.com/Portals/0/RPS%20document%20library/Open%20access/
Professional%20standards/Prescribing%20competency%20framework/
prescribing-competency-framework.pdf. Accessed 11 June 2017

WAG (2009) A community Nursing Strategy for Wales, Consultation
Document. Welsh Assembly Government, Cardiff

WAG (2010) Delivering a Five-Year Service, Workforce and Financial
Strategic Framework for NHS Wales. Welsh Assembly Government,
Cardiff

Welsh Assembly Government (2002) Improving health in Wales: remedies
for success—a strategy for pharmacy in Wales—a consultation document. Welsh Assembly Government, Cardiff

Welsh Assembly Government (2003) Review of health and social care in
Wales. The report of the project team advised by Derek Wanless. Welsh
Assembly Government, Cardiff

Welsh Assembly Government (WAG) (2005) Designed for life. Creating
world class health and social care for Wales in the 21st century. Welsh
Assembly Government, Cardiff

Welsh Government (2011) Together for health. A five year vision for the NHS in Wales. Welsh Government, Cardiff

Welsh Government (2015) Non-medical prescribing in Wales. Guidance. Welsh Government, Cardiff. Available via http://www.awmsg.org/docs/awmsg/medman/Non%20Medical%20Prescribing%20in%20Wales%20Guidance%202015.pdf. Accessed 11 Jun 2017

Welsh Statutory Instruments (2010) The National Health Service (miscellaneous amendments relating to independent prescribing) (Wales) regulations 2010 No.1647 (W.155). Available via https://legislation.vlex.co.uk/vid/miscellaneous-amendments-prescribing-338196926. Accessed 11 Jun 2017

# Chapter 4
# Non-medical Prescribing in Northern Ireland

**F. Lloyd, C.G. Adair, J. Agnew, C. Blayney, G. Boyd-McMurtry, O. Brown, A. Campbell, K. Clarke, P. Crawford, D. Gill, C. Harrison, J. McClelland, M.F. McManus, M. McMullan, B. Moore, R. O'Hare, L. O'Loan, M. Tennyson, and H. Winning**

------------

F. Lloyd (✉) • L. O'Loan
Assistant Director, NI Centre for Pharmacy Learning and Development,
Queen's University Belfast, Riddel Hall, 185 Stranmillis Road, Belfast
BT9 5EE, NI
e-mail: f.lloyd@qub.ac.uk

C.G. Adair
Director, NI Centre for Pharmacy Learning and Development,
Queen's University Belfast, Riddel Hall, 185 Stranmillis Road, Belfast
BT9 5EE, NI

C. Harrison
Senior Principal Pharmaceutical Officer, Department of Health,
Castle Buildings, Stormont, Belfast BT43SQ, NI

M.F. McManus
Nursing Officer, Department of Health, Castle Buildings, Stormont,
Belfast BT43SQ, NI

H. Winning
AHP Lead officer, Department of Health, Castle Buildings, Stormont,
Belfast BT43SQ, NI

C. Blayney
Pharmacy Adviser, Health and Social Care Board, Belfast, NI

G. Boyd-McMurtry
Medicines Management Co-ordinator, Health and Social Care Board,
Belfast, NI

© Springer International Publishing AG 2017
P.M. Franklin (ed.), *Non-medical Prescribing in the United Kingdom*,
DOI 10.1007/978-3-319-53324-7_4

53

M. McMullan
Clinical Optometric Adviser, Health and Social Care Board, Belfast, NI

O. Brown
Nurse Consultant of Service Development, Service Improvement, Public
Health Agency, Belfast, NI

M. Tennyson
Assistant Director Allied Health Professions & Personal and Public
Involvement, Public Health Agency, Belfast, NI

J. Agnew
Clinical Pharmacy Manager, Southern Health & Social Care Trust, Belfast, NI

A. Campbell
Clinical Pharmacy Development Lead, South Eastern Health & Social
Care Trust , Belfast,NI

K. Clarke
Lecturer in Podiatry, School of Health Sciences, Ulster University, Belfast, NI

J. McClelland
Lecturer in Optometry, School of Biomedical Sciences, Ulster University,
Belfast, NI

P. Crawford
Lead Clinical Pharmacist, Musgrave Park Hospital, Belfast Health &
Social Care Trust, Belfast, NI

D. Gill
Deputy Head Pharmacy and Medicines Management, Northern Health &
Social Care Trust, Belfast, NI

B. Moore
Clinical Pharmacy Manager, Western Health & Social Care Trust, Belfast, NI

R. O'Hare
Clinical Pharmacist, Queen's University,  Belfast, NI

**Abstract** The legislative changes needed to introduce
non-medical prescribing (NMP) in Northern Ireland (NI)
involve both UK wide legislation and NI Regulations.
Resultantly, some timing differences exist in the adoption of NMP legislation between GB and NI to allow
the devolved administration to adopt relevant legislation
locally. This Chapter considers the development of the local
legislation in terms of supplementary and independent

NMP with respect to pharmacists, nurses, physiotherapists, podiatrists, radiographers and optometrists.

A summary of the current prescribing status of each profession in NI is outlined by members of those professions. This highlights the progression of NMP across the professions, with several hundred pharmacists and nurses qualified and registered as NMPs, and the more recent professions to gain prescribing rights, such as optometrists, where fewer than 20 are currently registered as NMPs in NI. However, it is acknowledged that qualification and registration alone are not indicators of NMP activity and benefits and so the key achievements of active prescribers are considered where possible.

The Chapter concludes positively with an outline of what the future of NMP in NI may entail for each of those professions.

**Keywords**   Pharmacists • Physiotherapists • Podiatrists • Optometrists • Nurses • Northern Ireland • Governance • Prescribing • Non-medical prescribing

## 4.1   Introduction

Northern Ireland is a constituent unit of the United Kingdom (UK) of Great Britain (GB) and Northern Ireland (NI). It has a population of around 1.86 million (Northern Ireland Statistics and Research Agency 2016), constituting about 30% of the island of Ireland's total population and about 3% of the UK's population (Office for National Statistics 2016). The NI Assembly was established by the NI Act 1998, as part of the Good Friday Agreement, and is the devolved legislature for NI. It does not hold full legislative control of NI, just legislative control over certain matters, known as 'transferred matters', one of which is Health and Social Services (Cabinet office & Northern Ireland Office 2013).

NI has its own Department of Health (formerly known as the Department of Health, Social Services and Public Safety, DHSSPSNI), which is the government body responsible for Health and Social Care, including policy and legislation for hospitals, family practitioner services and community health and personal social services. In addition to this the NI Department of Health is also responsible for Public Health and Public Safety.

The NI Assembly has established a number of committees to oversee this legislative control. In the case of Health and Social Services, the Health Committee undertakes a scrutiny, policy development and consultation role with respect to the Department for Health and plays a key role in the consideration and development of legislation (Northern Ireland Assembly 2016). The legislative changes needed to introduce non-medical prescribing in NI involve both UK wide legislation and NI Regulations. Resultantly, some timing differences exist in the adoption of non-medical prescribing (NMP) legislation between GB and NI to allow the devolved administration to adopt relevant legislation locally and this is outlined, as appropriate, under each of the professions below.

Despite a devolved administration in NI, all health professions are regulated UK wide, with the exception of pharmacy. Pharmacy is unique in the UK in having two regulators, one regulating GB (General Pharmaceutical Council, GPhC) and one regulating NI (Pharmaceutical Society of Northern Ireland, PSNI). This has implications for the curriculum, training and accreditation of prescribing courses for pharmacists as outlined under this profession.

Nurse prescribing in various forms has been on the health agenda since 1986 and implemented in NI through a phased roll-out for district nurses and health visitors from 1999. The training programme in NI started in 2001 culminating in community practitioner nurse prescribers, whilst acting as independent prescribers could only prescribe from a limited formulary. Since 2003 nursing adopted extended nurse prescribing (later renamed supplementary and independent nurse prescribing). Therefore, whilst all other non-medical professions began their prescribing journeys with supplementary, developing into independent prescribing, it should be noted that nursing in all parts of the UK began with independent prescribing (albeit from a limited formulary).

However, this has been discussed previously in earlier chapters, and thus this chapter considers the progress since 2003 in relation to the roll-out of supplementary and then independent prescribing to the professions of pharmacy, optometry and the allied health professions (AHPs) of physiotherapy, podiatry and radiography, as applicable to NI. It also considers the further extension of prescribing rights (supplementary and independent) to the nursing profession in NI.

The history of the local legislation is charted with the implications on curriculum and training, followed by a summary of the current prescribing status of each profession. The Chapter concludes with an outline of what the future of non-medical prescribing (NMP) in NI may entail.

## 4.2   Supplementary Prescribing

On November 21st 2002, Lord Hunt announced new powers that would allow pharmacists and nurses in England to prescribe a wide range of drugs from 2003, through supplementary prescribing. In NI, the extension of supplementary prescribing rights to pharmacists was achieved through Article 47 of the Health and Personal Social Services (Quality, Improvement and Regulation) (NI) Order 2003 and to nurses through Article 3 of the Pharmaceutical Services (NI) Order 1992 (Department of Health, Social Services and Public Safety 2004). Supplementary prescribing is defined as 'a voluntary partnership between the independent prescriber and a supplementary prescriber, to implement an agreed patient-specific clinical management plan with the patient's agreement'. The clinical management plan (CMP) is the foundation stone of supplementary prescribing.

Before supplementary prescribing can take place, it is obligatory for an agreed CMP to be in place (written or electronic) relating to a named patient and to that patient's specific condition(s) to be managed by the supplementary prescriber (Department of Health 2003, 2005a, b; Department of Health, Social Services and Public Safety 2004). Supplementary prescribers must prescribe in partnership with a doctor or dentist, who is referred to as the independent prescriber.

## 4.3   Curriculum and Training

*Pharmacists*

The curriculum to train pharmacist supplementary prescribers in NI was developed by the then Royal Pharmaceutical Society of Great Britain (RPSGB) and the Pharmaceutical Society of Northern Ireland (PSNI), and pharmacists who wished to become a supplementary prescriber had to complete an accredited training programme. This entailed at least 25 days of training and an additional 12 days of learning in practice supervised by a medical practitioner, who is also known as a mentor. This curriculum is now obsolete and has been replaced by the outline curriculum to prepare pharmacists as both supplementary and independent prescribers (Royal Pharmaceutical Society of Great Britain 2006a, b; General Pharmaceutical Council 2016).

Currently, the only accredited provider of supplementary prescribing for pharmacists in NI is the Northern Ireland Centre for Pharmacy Learning and Development (NICPLD), School of Pharmacy, Queen's University Belfast. This course is accredited by both the GPhC and PSNI so that any pharmacists qualified as prescribers in NI can practise anywhere in the UK.

In NI, the first pharmacists from hospital practice enrolled on a supplementary prescribing training course on November 1st 2003 and the first community and primary care pharmacists enrolled on

March 1st 2004. Subsequently, the first 20 hospital pharmacist prescribers qualified in June 2004 and the first eight community/ primary care pharmacist prescribers qualified in December 2004.

*Nurses*

Nursing educational standards are set, and courses must be approved by the Nursing and Midwifery Council (NMC) all across the UK, including NI. Whilst programmes existed before 2003 to train nurses as community practitioner nurse prescribers (CPNPs), the legislation that allows nurses to become supplementary prescribers came into force in NI in 2003. In NI, courses to train nurses as supplementary prescribers comprised the equivalent of 600-h/75-day study, including at least 10 days of training at a university and an additional 15 days of learning in practice supervised by a medical practitioner, who is also known as a mentor (Department of Health, Social Services and Public Safety 2004).

The NMC set the standards for NMP. Since 2003, the accredited providers of independent and supplementary prescribing training in NI are Queen's University Belfast and Ulster University. In the nursing sector, the first nurses in NI were qualified as supplementary prescribers in 2003.

*Allied Health Professionals (Physiotherapists, Podiatrists or Chiropodists and Radiographers)*

In NI, on April 14, 2005, supplementary prescribing authority was extended to registered chiropodists and podiatrists, physiotherapists and radiographers (diagnostic and therapeutic) (Department of Health 2005b).

Despite the extension of supplementary prescribing rights to podiatrists, physiotherapists and radiographers in 2005, due to devolved legislative processes, no educational programmes emerged in NI for allied health professionals (AHPs) until 2009, when the training was commissioned by DHSSPSNI through

Ulster University, approved and accredited by the Health and Care Professions Council (HCPC).

The 2009 Postgraduate Certificate in Prescribing for AHPs comprised two 30 credit point modules, in combination leading to the award of Postgraduate Certificate in Prescribing for Allied Health Professionals and the professional award of supplementary prescribing (for those professions eligible). The design of the programme was underpinned by the Department of Health Outline Curriculum (Department of Health 2004).

The programme was a maximum of one academic year in duration. The programme was offered only as a part-time option with students expected to devote 78 h in clinical practice with a designated medical practitioner (DMP) as mentor to develop the requisite prescribing skills and competencies.

In NI, the first cohort comprising of two podiatrists, three therapeutic radiographers and six physiotherapists graduated in 2011.

### Optometrists

In NI, on April 14, 2005, supplementary prescribing authority was extended to registered chiropodists and podiatrists, physiotherapists, radiographers (diagnostic and therapeutic) and optometrists (Department of Health 2005b). In NI there are no training courses available for optometrists to train as a supplementary prescriber only.

## 4.4   Scope of Practice

Nurse and pharmacist supplementary prescribers are able to prescribe any medicine including controlled drugs, other than schedule 1 (since 2005). Supplementary prescribers may also prescribe medicines for use outside their licenced indications (off label) and unlicenced medicines that are part of a clinical trial, which have a clinical trial certificate or exemption and that are listed in an agreed clinical management plan (CMP) (Department of Health 2005b).

In NI, like other parts of the UK, all AHP and optometrist supplementary prescribers can prescribe any medicine, including controlled drugs, for any condition within their competence, the scope of supplementary prescribing being agreed within a patient's CMP, and for the medical judgement of the independent prescribers as to the appropriateness of the plan and its agreement.

## 4.5 Independent Prescribing

Whilst nurses already had achieved prescribing rights, the extension of prescribing rights to pharmacists in 2003 was hailed as a major advancement for the pharmacy profession and as a logical next step in the move towards a more patient-centred profession. The RPSGB warmly welcomed the introduction of supplementary prescribing by pharmacists and the government's progress on implementation and expected that this would pave the way for the introduction of independent pharmacist prescribing (Royal Pharmaceutical Society of Great Britain 2003; Anon 2005). Following a joint Medicines and Healthcare Products Regulatory Agency (MHRA) and Department of Health consultation in 2005, independent prescribing by nurses and pharmacists was enabled when the UK-wide Medicines and Human Use (Prescribing) (Miscellaneous Amendments) Order was changed in May 2006. Further amendments to regulations put these changes into effect in NI from August 2006 (Department of Health, Social Services and Public Safety 2006). The Department of Health's definition of independent prescribing was 'prescribing by a practitioner (e.g. doctor, dentist, nurse, pharmacist) who is responsible and accountable for the assessment of patients with undiagnosed or diagnosed conditions and for decisions about the clinical management required, including prescribing' (Department of Health, Social Services and Public Safety 2006; Department of Health 2006).

## 4.6 Curriculum and Training

*Pharmacists*

Since 2006, any pharmacists who wish to become prescribers (either supplementary or independent) must complete an accredited programme. Independent prescribing programmes comprise of at least 26 days of teaching, with an additional 12 days of learning in practice supervised by a medical practitioner, also known as a mentor (Royal Pharmaceutical Society of Great Britain 2006a).

Pharmacist supplementary prescribers who have been qualified as a prescriber for less than 5 years can become independent prescribers by completing a conversion course. The conversion course involves the equivalent of 2 days' didactic learning and a minimum of 2 days' learning in practice supervised by a medical practitioner (mentor) (Royal Pharmaceutical Society of Great Britain 2006b). The first 29 independent prescribing pharmacists in NI qualified in March 2007 by virtue of a conversion course.

Since March 2007 the only accredited course (GPhC/PSNI) available to pharmacists in NI is a combined supplementary and independent prescribing course (NICPLD 2016, Personal communication).

*Nurses*

Whilst other non-medical professions began their prescribing journeys with supplementary and then independent prescribing,

**Table 4.1**  List of prescribing qualifications available to nurses in NI (NB, this is the same as for England and Scotland)

| Programme code | Qualification |
|---|---|
| V100 | Community practitioner nurse prescriber |
| V150 | Community practitioner nurse prescriber (without specialist practice qualification or specialist community public health nurse) |
| V200 | Extended formulary nurse prescriber |
| V300 | Nurse independent/supplementary prescribing |

For information concerning Wales, please see chapter on Non-medical Prescribing in Wales

nurses have been able to prescribe independently in various forms since 2001. Whilst programmes still exist to train as community practitioner nurse prescribers (CPNPs), successful candidates are limited to a nurse prescriber's formulary. Currently, in NI, the only NMC-accredited full non-medical prescribing course available to nurses in NI is a combined supplementary and independent prescribing course (leading to annotation on NMC register) (Table 4.1).

The first nurses in NI to qualify as independent and supplementary prescribers through the V300 route were in 2003.

*Optometrists*

In August 2007, the Department of Health in NI announced that optometrists would be able to train to prescribe medicines as independent prescribers (Department of Health, Social Services and Public Safety 2008a).

Independent prescribing training for optometrists is not NI specific. There are currently four courses in the UK (Ulster University, Glasgow Caledonian, City University London and Aston/Manchester joint programme) where qualified optometrists, registered with the General Optical Council (GOC), may undertake the theoretical part of the programme. The curriculum is set and courses are accredited and monitored by GOC, the regulatory body for optometrists in the UK. Currently, the only accredited provider of the theoretical component of optometrist independent prescribing training in NI is Ulster University. The accredited course at Ulster University consists of two 30 credit online modules comprising weekly lectures, weekly multiple choice questionnaires and three additional pieces of coursework per module.

The theoretical component of the course is then followed by 24 half-day hospital sessions under the supervision of an ophthalmologist. This part of the training is managed and administered by the College of Optometrists. After the clinical placement, optometrists are required to take the professional examination, set by the College of Optometrists, known as the Common Final Assessment in Therapeutics. Once an optometrist passes the final professional examination, they may apply to join a specialist GOC register.

The first optometrist independent prescribers were qualified in 2009 in GB. To date, there are no optometrist independent prescribers working in NI who have qualified from an NI-based course, as the only accredited course (Ulster University) began in January 2016 with the first graduates starting their clinical placements from April 2017 (McClelland 2016, Personal communication). However, according to the GOC register, there are 16 independent prescribing optometrists registered in NI (General Optical Council 2016). Those optometrists undertook their training in GB but practise in NI.

### Allied Health Professionals (Physiotherapists, Podiatrists or Chiropodists and Radiographers)

UK-wide changes to legislation to enable the introduction of independent prescribing by physiotherapists and podiatrists or chiropodists were announced by the Department of Health on

July 24, 2012, and subsequent changes by DHSSPSNI to regulations came into force in NI on July 18, 2014, to allow the dispensing against prescriptions issued by physiotherapists and podiatrists or chiropodists who have qualified as independent prescribers (Department of Health, Social Services and Public Safety 2015b).

In recognition of the legislative change and with the Department of Health, NI, being the primary driver, the previous part-time Postgraduate Certificate was modified to include independent prescribing competencies in alignment with competency frameworks for the same from the Department of Health, the HCPC and the National Prescribing Centre. A further conversion programme was also developed to allow those with legislative rights who met the required criteria to upgrade from supplementary to independent prescriber status and the current 'Medicines Management Framework' emerged.

Currently, Ulster University is the only accredited provider of independent and supplementary prescriber training for podiatrists and physiotherapists and supplementary prescriber training for radiographers in NI.

The AHP independent and/or supplementary prescriber training consists of a minimum of 38 days, within which students should undertake a minimum of 26 days' theoretical learning and a minimum of 90 hours practice-based learning with a designated medical practitioner (DMP) or mentor (Allied Health Professions Federation 2013a). AHP supplementary prescribers who have been qualified 6 months or greater and are practising prescribers can train to become an independent prescriber by completing the short conversion programme comprising a minimum 2 days didactic learning and 2 days learning in clinical practice with a DMP (Allied Health Professions Federation 2013b).

The first cohort of Independent Prescriber AHPs in NI graduated via the Medicines Management (conversion to independent prescribing) programme at Ulster University in 2014 and comprised 3 podiatrists and 11 physiotherapists.

Since February 2016 therapeutic radiographers are able to qualify as independent prescribers in England. The administrations in NI, Scotland and Wales will decide whether to adopt the same practice (Mawhinney 2016, Personal communication).

## 4.7 Scope of Practice

From 2006, suitably trained independent prescribing pharmacists and independent prescribing nurses can prescribe any licenced medicine, with the exception of controlled drugs in the case of pharmacists until 2012, for any medical condition within their competence. They can prescribe medicines outside their licenced indications (off label) where this is an accepted clinical practice (Department of Health 2006; Department of Health, Social Services and Public Safety 2006). Since 2010, following an MHRA public consultation earlier in the year (proposal for amendments to medicines legislation to allow mixing of medicines in palliative care), changes to legislation have come into force to allow nurse and pharmacist independent prescribers in NI to prescribe unlicenced medicines (Department of Health, Social Services and Public Safety 2015a).

Up until 2008, nurse independent prescribers were authorised to prescribe some specific controlled drugs but only for specified medical conditions (Department of Health, Social Services and Public Safety 2008b). Amendments to the Misuse of Drugs Regulations (Northern Ireland) 2002 introduced on May 10, 2012, allowed nurse independent prescribers and pharmacist independent prescribers in NI to prescribe any controlled drugs in Schedules 2–5 (Department of Health, Social Services and Public Safety 2012a).

Optometrist prescribers can prescribe any licenced medicine (non-parenteral) for ocular conditions affecting the eye and surrounding tissue, but are not authorised to prescribe any controlled drugs (Department of Health, Northern Ireland 2016a).

Physiotherapists, podiatrists and chiropodists independent prescribers can prescribe drugs, which fall within their area of competence, and since June 2015 in England, Scotland and Wales, they can prescribe a specific, limited group of controlled drugs (Chartered Society of Physiotherapy 2016). In NI, physiotherapists, podiatrists and chiropodists cannot currently independently prescribe any controlled drugs. Legislation in NI is currently being amended with changes expected in 2017 (Mawhinney 2016, Personal communication).

## 4.8 Current Status in Primary and Secondary Care for Pharmacist Prescribers

Between 2003 and 2016, 303 pharmacists in NI have qualified as either a supplementary and/or an independent prescriber. The majority ($n = 293$) are qualified as both supplementary and independent prescribers, with only a few pharmacists ($n = 10$) choosing not to convert their supplementary qualification to an independent qualification when the conversion course was offered (2006–2009). Of the total number qualified, just over two-thirds are from the hospital sector [205/303 (67.6%)] and almost one-third [98/303 (32.3%)] from the community or primary care sectors.

Table 4.2 documents the broad range of clinical areas that pharmacists in NI underwent in their training in 2003–2016. From Table 4.2 it can be seen that the largest proportion of pharmacists undergoing training specified their clinical area as that of a generalist, managing patients with multiple morbidities. The move to the role of a generalist was driven by the heads of pharmacy and medicines management in the five hospital trusts across NI who felt a more generalist prescriber would be more useful to the hospital as they can work in general areas such as medical or surgical admissions and care of the elderly wards. This broader approach avoids duplicating the work of nursing

**Table 4.2** List of clinical areas pharmacists specified whilst undertaking pharmacist prescribing training course in NI (2003–2015)

| Clinical area | No. of pharmacists trained | Percentage of total (%) |
| --- | --- | --- |
| Antimicrobial therapy, cardiovascular disease, respiratory disease, diabetes (generalist hospital prescribers) | 48 | 15.8 |
| Hypertension (including chronic kidney disease) | 37 | 12.2 |
| Anticoagulation | 30 | 9.9 |
| Cardiovascular risk management (hypertension and associated risk factors) | 26 | 8.5 |
| Asthma/COPD/respiratory disease | 21 | 6.9 |
| Renal medicine | 19 | 6.3 |
| Diabetes (including cardiovascular risk reduction) | 18 | 5.9 |
| Pain management | 13 | 4.2 |
| Antimicrobial prescribing | 12 | 3.9 |
| Haematology/oncology | 11 | 3.6 |
| Benzodiazepine reduction/clinical addiction/substance misuse/alcohol withdrawal | 9 | 2.9 |
| Secondary prevention of stroke | 6 | 1.9 |
| Management of obesity | 5 | 1.6 |
| Paediatric renal medicine/respiratory/ asthma/epilepsy/pain management/ rheumatology/general | 5 | 1.6 |
| Elderly care | 4 | 1.3 |
| Critical care (ICU and TPN) | 4 | 1.3 |
| Rheumatology | 4 | 1.3 |
| Oncology and paediatric oncology | 4 | 1.3 |
| Cardiology (pulmonary hypertension) | 3 | 0.9 |
| Gastroenterology | 3 | 0.9 |
| Osteoporosis—prevention and treatment | 3 | 0.9 |
| Dermatology | 2 | 0.6 |
| Cellulitis | 2 | 0.6 |

**Table 4.2**   (continued)

| Clinical area | No. of pharmacists trained | Percentage of total (%) |
|---|---|---|
| Palliative care | 2 | 0.6 |
| Orthopaedics | 2 | 0.6 |
| HIV/infectious diseases | 2 | 0.6 |
| Atopic disease—eczema, asthma, allergies | 1 | 0.3 |
| Menopause clinic | 1 | 0.3 |
| Endocarditis | 1 | 0.3 |
| Depression | 1 | 0.3 |
| Psychiatry | 1 | 0.3 |
| Parkinson's disease | 1 | 0.3 |
| Heart failure | 1 | 0.3 |
| Total | 303 | |

Source: NICPLD (2016)

and medical colleagues who tend to work in more narrow, specialised areas. However, some pharmacists only work in specialised areas (e.g. renal, oncology), and in some cases the clinical pharmacy manager decided it was not appropriate for them to train as a generalist prescriber.

*Secondary Care*

Up until 2016, the only pharmacists to opt for the role of a generalist prescriber were hospital pharmacists. To explain the justification for hospital generalist prescribers, the head of pharmacy and medicines management in one of the five hospital trusts states:

> *The majority of our non-medical prescribers are generic pharmacist independent prescribers. This allows us to utilise their skills as part of their daily work on the ward rather than the original prescribers who set up outpatient clinics but were never backfilled and so created issues with ward cover.*

*The pharmacists are based in Emergency Department, Minor Ailments Unit, medical wards and one surgical ward. Using generic treatment plans they can use their Pharmacist Independent Prescriber skills to ensure the medicines kardex is correct from admission and during their inpatient stay. They use their skills primarily during the medicines reconciliation process ensuring the medicines prescribed are optimised for each individual patient. Ensuring the kardex is correct as close to admission as possible minimises any patient safety issues and omitted doses.* (Head of Pharmacy and Medicines Management June 8, 2016)

This is reiterated by a clinical pharmacy manager in a different trust:

*We are using more of our prescribers as generalist prescribers. Many of them did not originally train as a generalist but have moved to this. Presently they are working in Trauma and Orthopaedics and some of our medical wards. They are able to resolve prescribing omissions and errors at admission and discharge. This reduces delayed and omitted medicines and speeds up the discharge process. The pharmacists in Trauma and Orthopaedics prescribe enoxaparin for outpatients with lower limb casts until their fracture clinic appointment ensuring that anticoagulant therapy is continued minimising the risk of VTE. Working as a generalist prescriber helps to improve relationships with medical staff as many of the prescribing issues that medical staff perceive as minor can now be dealt with by a pharmacist. It also gives the pharmacist generalist prescriber greater job satisfaction.* (Clinical Pharmacy Manager 13th June 2016)

Reflective of the areas that pharmacists underwent training in, pharmacists in hospital practice in NI prescribe in a broad range of clinical areas/wards. Table 4.3 documents a summary of the clinical areas/wards, which pharmacist prescribers are working across in the five hospital trusts in NI (current June 2016).

## Governance Arrangements in Secondary Care

In addition to the standard governance arrangements in secondary care, each trust in NI has a NMP committee and a non-medical prescribing governance framework. The framework

**Table 4.3** Summary of pharmacist prescribing status in secondary care in NI, June 2016

| Hospital trust | No. qualified pharmacist prescribers | Clinical area/ward |
|---|---|---|
| 1 | 37 (27 practising, 10 not practising) | Paediatrics, anticoagulation, antibiotics, trauma and orthopaedics, accident and emergency, cardiovascular, renal, TPN, stroke, care of the elderly and palliative care |
| 2 | 26 (21 practising, 5 not practising) | Generalist prescribers covering cardiovascular, diabetes, antimicrobial and respiratory<br>Other specialist areas covered are renal, diabetes, cancer, care of older people, gastroenterology, acute care at home, ICU/HD, anticoagulation and antimicrobials |
| 3 | 26 (division between practising/not practising unavailable) | Renal, diabetes, diabetes cardiovascular risk prevention, antibiotics, acute admissions, cancer, care of older people, respiratory, gastroenterology, acute care at home, ICU/HD, warfarin/anticoagulants |
| 4 | 37 (34 practising, 3 not practising) | 25 generalist prescribers covering cardiovascular, diabetes, antimicrobial and respiratory, working to trust treatment plan for pharmacist NMP<br>Other specialist areas covered are renal, haematology, rheumatology, menopause, anticoagulation, critical care and surgery |
| 5 | 32 (17 practising, 15 not practising) | Generalist prescribers covering cardiovascular, diabetes, antimicrobial and respiratory<br>Other specialist areas covered are cardiology, anticoagulation, diabetes, elderly care, HIV/GUM, mental health, pain, paediatrics, renal, respiratory and antimicrobials, rheumatology, surgical, vascular and admissions |

Source: NMP Pharmacy Lead in five Hospital Trusts across NI

applies to all registered practitioners who are registered non-medical prescribers including registered nurses, registered pharmacists and registered AHPs. The framework aims to promote patient/client safety and reduce risks associated with medicines management and to ensure NMP staff are supported in their professional practice.

The requirement for pharmacist prescribing must be implicit in the job description for the pharmacist to ensure that the trust indemnity will protect both patients and the staff member.

In NI, pharmacists in secondary care only prescribe on medical records (Kardex) or outpatient letters and hence have no impact on the NMP budget. The NMP budget covers prescribing by NMPs who are employed in secondary care but see patients in primary care, e.g. district nurses and optometrists.

### Community/Primary Care Sector

The majority of community/primary care pharmacists tended to specialise in one clinical area (e.g. hypertension) as their area of expertise whilst undergoing training.

Between 2007 and 2016, qualified pharmacist prescribers could apply for funding to prescribe in a primary care setting. The funding was limited to a maximum of 38 sessions/year (including two training sessions). Pharmacists were paid a fee of £150/session. Prescribing had to be supported by the GP practice and in line with the Pharmaceutical Clinical Effectiveness (PCE) programme from the Health Social Care Board (HSCB), NI, available via https://www.health-ni.gov.uk/articles/pharmaceutical-clinical-effectiveness-programme, accessed on December 30, 2016.

Even taking into account that the clinical area pharmacist chose to prescribe in were restrained by the PCE clinical areas, overall, the range of clinical area pharmacists in community/primary care sector actually prescribed in tended to be narrower than the hospital sector. The clinical area chosen by pharmacists in community/primary care tended to centre on hypertension.

However, the number of clinical areas selected by any one prescriber tended to increase over time as their experience and confidence grew. For example, a prescriber may have started out in hypertension only but added hyperlipidaemia the following year and cardiovascular risk the year after that. Table 4.4 shows the range of clinical areas for which 40 pharmacist prescribers were funded in the year 2015–2016.

**Table 4.4** Summary of clinical areas for which pharmacist prescribers in primary care in NI were funded in 2015–2016

| Clinical area | No. pharmacists funded 2015–2016 |
|---|---|
| Hypertension and hyperlipidaemia | 14 |
| Cardiovascular risk reduction | 3 |
| Pain | 3 |
| Asthma | 2 |
| Hypertension | 2 |
| Hypertension, hyperlipidaemia and cardiovascular risk | 2 |
| Cardiovascular and benzodiazepine reduction | 1 |
| Hypertension, hyperlipidaemia and osteoporosis | 1 |
| Respiratory, hypertension, hyperlipidaemia and acute | 1 |
| Diabetes and hypertension | 1 |
| Hypertension and CKD | 1 |
| Medication review: elderly and nursing home | 1 |
| Hypertension and acute prescribing | 1 |
| Hypertension and chronic non-cancer pain | 1 |
| Cardiovascular and diabetes | 1 |
| Cardiovascular and proton pump inhibitors | 1 |
| Hypertension, rheumatology, asthma review, nursing home and acute | 1 |
| Hypertension and benzodiazepine review | 1 |
| COPD and asthma | 1 |
| Respiratory | 1 |
| Total | 40 |

Source: HSCB

**Table 4.5** Summary of clinical areas for which pharmacist prescribers in primary care in NI were funded in 2016–2017

| Clinical area | No. pharmacists funded 2016–2017 |
| --- | --- |
| Cardiovascular | 24 (45%) |
| Generalist | 14 (26%) |
| Respiratory | 7 (13%) |
| Pain | 4 (8%) |
| Other (PPI reduction, type 2 diabetes, CKD and care of the elderly) | 4 (8%) |
| Total | 53 |

Source: HSCB

In 2016–2017 the HSCB funded 53 pharmacist independent prescribers (increase of 47% since 2012–2013) to run clinics in 56 GP surgeries across NI. Table 4.5 shows the clinical areas for which the 53 pharmacists were funded in 2016–2017. Since 2012, pharmacists have been developing and expanding their competence to enable them to work in a generalist capacity, which is clearly demonstrated by the large number now working in a generalist role (i.e. across two or more therapeutic areas such as cardiovascular and respiratory) in 2016–2017. Many of these generalists are responsible for the acute and repeat prescription systems within their GP surgeries.

*Primary Care: Nursing Home Reviews*

In 2013, the Pharmacist Nursing Home Medication Review Initiative aligned 31 pharmacist prescribers with 32 GP surgeries in NI. The pharmacist prescribers reviewed the medication of 1130 nursing home patients (approx. 10% of NI nursing home population), making a total of 3807 interventions (2392 prescribing interventions and 1415 non-prescribing interventions). It is estimated that the annual cost savings associated with the 2392 prescribing interventions was £213,000.

In terms of the potential of pharmacist prescriber nursing home medication reviews, it is clear that prescribers were extremely effective in undertaking these reviews, yielding both health benefits to the nursing home residents whilst realising substantial prescribing savings and indirect savings for the HSC through more cost-effective and appropriate prescribing (Blayney 2016, Personal communication).

## Primary Care: Out of Hours Pilot

In 2015, eight pharmacist prescribers were involved in an inno-vative 6-month pilot in the Southern Health and Social Care Trust. The eight pharmacist prescribers were embedded within GP out of hours (OOH) to help manage demand. Prescribers worked 5 hour shifts at periods of highest demand (Saturday/Sunday and Public Holidays). The pharmacists' priority was to deal with requests for repeat medications and then to enter the general triage and deal with cases for the treatment of minor acute conditions within their competence, e.g. morning after pill, impetigo, cold sores, uncomplicated urinary tract infec-tions, coughs and colds, etc. During the 61 × 5 hour shifts, pharmacists closed 895 cases of the 10,714 cases entering the system during that time. This averaged out as 14.6 cases closed per shift and approximately 9% of the overall demand on the service. The pilot was extended for another year and plans are being made to commission this service regionally in the future.

## Governance Arrangements in Primary Care

Pharmacists in primary care in NI prescribe only in the GP set-ting (with exception of nursing home/out of hours pilots). Pharmacist prescribers are required to register with the NI NMP Electronic Registration Database, which collates information on employer details, qualifications and parameters of prescribing. The database generates a four-digit cipher number, which links the pharmacist to the practice they are working in (attributing their prescribing to the primary care budget, not NMP budget) and allows monitoring of prescribing. All prescribing by NMPs is monitored on a quarterly basis to ensure it reflects the parameters of prescribing on the registration database.

## 4.9  Current Status in Primary and Secondary Care for Nurse Prescribers

The number of nurse prescribers in NI registered with the NMC August 2016 is detailed in Table 4.6.

Nurses in general practice and trust employed community nurses also have to register with their employers in order to practise as prescribers. Currently 475 nurses in NI are registered as independent and supplementary prescribers (Brown 2016, Personal communication). The variance can be explained by a number of reasons, e.g. retirement (many were the more senior experienced nurses), movement into management roles, working in hospital outpatient clinics and therefore recommending rather than prescribing.

**Table 4.6** Number of nurses qualified as prescribers and registered with NMC (current October 2016)

| Programme code | Type of nurse prescriber | Total number registered with NMC in NI |
|---|---|---|
| V100 | Community practitioner nurse prescriber | 1262 |
| V150 | Community practitioner nurse prescriber | 33 |
| V200 | Nurse independent prescriber | 1 |
| V300 | Nurse independent/supplementary prescriber | 644 |

*Governance Arrangements in Primary Care*

As with pharmacists, nurses are required to register with the NI NMP Electronic Registration Database, which facilitates monitoring of prescribing. Prior to the creation of a NMP budget, nurses working across numerous practices were required to have multiple prescription pads. The NMP budget has enabled nurses to have only one prescription pad for all clients and thus removed this barrier to prescribing (NIPEC 2014).

## 4.10 Current Status in Primary and Secondary Care for Optometrist Prescribers

According to the GOC register, there are 16 independent prescribing optometrists registered in NI available via https://www.optical.org/en/utilities/online-registers.cfm. Accessed 12th June 2017. Those independent prescribing optometrists working in NI have qualified in one of the other three courses in the UK (Glasgow Caledonian, City University London and Aston/Manchester joint programme).

Independent prescribing optometrists currently work in both the primary care setting as community optometrists and in the secondary care setting in hospital clinics. Whilst acknowledging that total numbers are small ($n = 16$), there is a slight majority working in the primary care setting. The scope of practice for independent prescribing hospital optometrists in NI is slowly changing with four independent prescribing optometrists recently having been recruited for eye casualty sessions, and there are three to four currently working in glaucoma clinics across the region (McMullan 2016, Personal communication).

Whilst still in its infancy in the hospital setting, benefits in efficiency and multidisciplinary team working are already being realised as described by the Head of Optometry in one of the five hospital trusts in NI:

*Optometrist Independent Prescribing is relatively new but is already making a huge impact to ophthalmic clinics within our Trust. The ability to manage patients to completion and alter treatments without requirement to consult with medical staff has greatly increased the efficiency of the clinics. These skills have been utilised in a number of high volume ophthalmic outpatient groups including glaucoma, pre and post-operative cataract, anterior segment and eye casualty clinics. IP Optometrists are suitably trained to enable a knowledgeable discussion on medications and their effects with patients, which also significantly improves the patient experience and understanding of their treatment.*

*Liaison with other independent prescribing professions via Trust Non-Medical Prescribing (NMP) groups has also been helpful in promoting shared learning, increasing safety and improving general understanding of independent prescribing pathways within the Trust.* (Head of Optometry, Health and Social Care Trust)

Independent prescribing optometrists in primary care can register with the HSCB as a non-medical prescriber and have access to HS21 prescription pads to enable issuing of Health and Social Care (HSC)-funded prescriptions. Independent prescribing community optometrists in the course of their clinical practice examine patients and determine if prescribing is the most appropriate course of action to manage the clinical presentation. Objective 10 of the Department of Health policy document *Developing Eyecare Partnerships, Improving the Commissioning and Provision of Eyecare Services in NI (October 2012)* (DEP) states:

*Clinical leadership, workforce development, training, supervision and accreditation will be essential components of eyecare service reform. This includes the promotion of independent optometrists' prescribing, where appropriate to do so.*

The work of the above has resulted in developments in the field of independent prescribing optometry. The HSCB has enabled optometrists in primary care to access HS21 prescription pads to allow patients to access their prescription for ophthalmic medication at source from the independent prescribing optometrist. In addition the HSCB is working with Health and Social Care Trusts to establish a framework whereby optometrists undertaking their training can access the necessary ophthalmic clinical sessions in secondary care. It is hoped that although numbers may be limited at the outset, this can be developed as outcomes are evaluated and capacity established. Currently there is no allocated training budget for optometrists to undertake their independent prescribing training and optometrists self-fund their training.

Independent prescribing optometrists working in primary care have skills, which add value to the patient pathway and experience. Objective 9 of DEPs provides direction for the HSCB to develop a regional pathway for patients who experience non-sight-threatening acute eye problems allowing them to be assessed, triaged and managed by primary care optometrists in the community setting (Department of Health, Social Services and Public Safety 2012b). The ability of independent prescribing optometrists, working in their community practices, to prescribe and treat patients where it is safe and appropriate to do so will add value to this pathway.

*Governance Arrangements in Primary Care*

The governance arrangements and monitoring of primary care-based independent prescribing optometrists are aligned to other primary care non-medical prescribers, e.g. pharmacists. Registration is undertaken and a non-medical prescriber induction is undertaken for all independent prescribing optometrists who wish to access HS21 prescription pads when working in primary care practice. Independent prescribing optometrists issue prescriptions within parameters defined by their competency. They can extend the parameters of prescribing and update their prescribing details as necessary. Monitoring of primary care independent prescribing optometrists is undertaken on a quarterly basis by a Prescribing Support Officer from HSCB with the type and level of prescribing activity being reviewed by HSCB ophthalmic clinical advisers.

## 4.11    Current Status in Primary and Secondary Care for Allied Health Professionals (Physiotherapist/Podiatrist or Chiropodist/ Radiographer)

To date, there have been 51 AHPs trained as independent and/ or supplementary prescribers in NI, 5 podiatrists, 3 therapeutic radiographers and 44 physiotherapists, all with varying specialisms and working in both primary and secondary care sectors.

Independent prescribing is considered optimal due to the clinical autonomy it provides for professionals already trained and competent in assessment and diagnosis of their own patient caseload. Supplementary prescribing has been demonstrated to work efficiently in the management of long-term conditions and in particular in secondary care and, however, has not been without the same limitations as those identified by other professions (e.g. time constraints imposed by the development and agreement of CMPs and restricted access to drugs within the plan).

Support from both the Department of Health, NI, and the Public Health Agency (PHA) has ensured that any issues around implementation are closely monitored and managed. Resultantly, there are very few AHPs trained in NI who are not currently prescribing.

*Governance Arrangements in Primary Care*

Currently the implementation of independent prescribing for physiotherapists and podiatrists is progressing; governance arrangements are in place in secondary care trusts, but there are local challenges for independent AHP NMPs in accessing the prescription pads (HS21) currently being used by other independent NMPs.

## 4.12 The Future of Non-medical Prescribing in NI

*Future in Primary Care for Pharmacist Prescribers*

Since 2007, pharmacist independent prescribers (PIP) have been funded to provide clinics in primary care in conjunction with a GP practice. The success of these clinics has influenced the development of a permanent role for pharmacists in general practice, and in 2016 the Department of Health announced a major investment programme for practice-based pharmacists in NI. The programme will employ practice-based pharmacists (PBP) in all GP practices in NI.

In acknowledging Northern Ireland's over-reliance on hospital care, *Transforming Your Care* (Department of Health, Social Services and Public Safety 2011) sets out a broad new model of care focused on supporting patient-centred care. Its most substantial proposal was to move £83 million from hospitals to primary, community and social care services. This policy recognised an enhanced role for pharmacy to support patient-centred care by helping people stay independent and well, gaining optimal benefits from their medicines. The expansion of the pharmacist's role into primary care is an important component of the Department of Health's Medicines Optimisation Quality Framework (MOQF). The MOQF supports an integrated approach to medicine optimisation with pharmacists working collaboratively in primary and secondary care and community pharmacy settings. The recent recruitment of pharmacist prescribers to every general medical practice in Northern Ireland is a practical solution to build capacity in primary care. It is anticipated that by April 2017 the full complement of pharmacists will be recruited to the GP federations who have been allocated with the funding for all pharmacist independent prescriber (PIP) services within primary care through the PBP model.

The PBP model marks a huge transformation in practice for pharmacists in NI. These pharmacists are expected to either be independent prescribing pharmacists or willing to undertake the qualification. As this new mode of practice is not yet established, it is unknown whether these prescribing pharmacists will be working in specialised clinic roles (e.g. hypertension) or working in a broader prescribing role (e.g. managing the repeat prescribing system). There is an expectation that there will be a progression within their prescribing role over time. A separate evaluation of this model will be taking place and available in due course.

### Future in Secondary Care for Pharmacist Prescribers

The 2001 Audit Commission report, *A Spoonful of Sugar* (Audit Commission 2001), considered the developing role of the pharmacy technicians as vital to freeing pharmacists from their supply function to focus on clinical roles. At the same time while NICPLD began training pharmacist prescribers, it also assumed responsibility for the post-qualification training of pharmacy technicians. NICPLD introduced the Accredited Checking Pharmacy Technician (ACPT) programme in 2002, and, as a result, the skill mix in hospital dispensaries has been transformed, with the majority of medicines supply functions now undertaken by pharmacy technicians enabling pharmacists to become more clinically focused.

All newly qualified pharmacists working in secondary care now undertake a structured work-based Foundation Programme, which focuses on implementing best practice in medicine optimisation, as recommended in the Medicines Optimisation Quality Framework (MOQF). Pharmacists completing the Foundation Programme are strongly encouraged to progress on to an Advanced Pharmacy Practice (APP) programme, which incorporates the prescribing qualification (Department of Health, Social Services and Public Safety 2010). Stage 1 of the APP programme enables pharmacists to qualify as generalist prescribers who can optimise and prescribe medicines for patients with multiple morbidities. Stage 2 helps pharmacists to manage more complex patients in specialist therapeutic areas (e.g. renal). Their generalist training in Stage 1 helps them to manage these complex specialist patients holistically and differentiates them from their medical and nursing colleagues who tend to prescribe in their specialist area only.

In addition, other plans incorporating pharmacist prescribers in secondary care include a consultant pharmacist led model for older people in intermediate care, care home and domiciliary care settings, prescribers in Emergency Departments and managing discharges.

An important element in the success of pharmacist prescribing in primary and secondary care in NI has been the close cooperation between policymakers, service commissioner, heads of pharmacy in the hospital trusts and the training provider. It is important to emphasise that prescribing is only one of the enabling skills for pharmacists. To be effective, it is envisaged that the primary care workforce should be developed along the same pathway as their hospital counterparts.

## Future in Primary and Secondary Care for Nurse Prescribers

Delivering Together (Department of Health, Northern Ireland 2016b) has set out the Minister's vision to transform Health and Social Care in NI. As part of the transformation in NI, there is a greater need to expand and fully utilise nurse prescribers within primary and secondary care, including out of hours nurse practitioners, development of advanced nurse practitioners, specialists nurses and General Practice nurses, to meet the needs of patients. Nurse Independent and Supplementary prescribing makes better use of the skills and knowledge of experienced nurses and improves patient care (NIPEC 2014).

## Future in Primary and Secondary Care for Optometrist Prescribers

As service developments implemented through the work of DEPs are expanded and rolled out, for example, the Southern Primary Eyecare Assessment and Referral Service (SPEARS) (Health and Social Care Board 2016), and the number of qualified independent prescribing optometrists in primary care community practices increases in NI, this will help manage demand on secondary care. The aim is to provide safe and timely access to eyecare service (patients assessed and were appropriately treated closer to home aligned to Transforming Your Care), thereby reducing the burden on busy eye casualty departments allowing ophthalmologists time to see more complex cases. In addition increased numbers and availability of independent prescribing optometrists in the community will improve antimicrobial stewardship ensuring that topical antibiotics are only prescribed when clinically indicated following appropriate clinical assessment.

In parallel, optometrists with this qualification will hopefully become more integrated into specialised hospital roles including glaucoma management. An increase in knowledge and skills will ensure that the standard of care that optometrists in NI provide for their patients will continue to improve and allows optometry to continue to develop professionally and in line with other countries.

*Future in Primary and Secondary Care for Allied Health
Professionals (Physiotherapist/Podiatrist/Radiographer)*

The future of AHP prescribing, whether independent, supplementary or by supportive mechanism such as the use of exemptions order process is strongly supported by the professions involved and the PHA, NI. Providing AHPs with the opportunity to prescribe significantly advances the care, skills and service the professions can provide and allows a more efficient and streamlined service, meaning the patient receives the medicines they require at point of care without compromise to safety.

In NI, there is further potential for AHP NMPs to work in the primary care setting, maximising their prescribing abilities. The potential for physiotherapists to work in primary care (GP practices) is being explored regionally and nationally and these clinicians would be ideally placed to optimise NMP skills.

# References

Allied Health Professions Federation, Chartered Society of Physiotherapy, Institute of Chiropodists and Podiatrists, The Society and College of Radiographers, The College of Podiatry (2013a) Outline curriculum framework for education programmes to prepare physiotherapists and podiatrists as independent/supplementary prescribers and to prepare radiographers as supplementary prescribers. Available via http://www.csp.org.uk/documents/outline-curriculum-framework-education-programmes-prepare-physiotherapists-podiatrists-ind

Allied Health Professions Federation, Chartered Society of Physiotherapy, Institute of Chiropodists and Podiatrists, The Society and College of Radiographers, The College of Podiatry (2013b) Outline curriculum framework for conversion programmes to prepare physiotherapist and podiatrist supplementary prescribers as independent prescribers. Available via http://www.csp.org.uk/documents/outline-curriculum-framework-conversion-programmes-prepare-physiotherapist-podiatrist-supp. Accessed 12 Jun 2017

Anon (2005) Pharmacist independent prescribing given go-ahead. Pharm J 275:621

Audit Commission (2001) A spoonful of sugar: medicines management in NHS hospitals. Available via http://www.eprescribingtoolkit.com/wp-content/uploads/2013/11/nrspoonfulsugar1.pdf. Accessed 21 Dec 2016

Blayney C (2016) Personal communication. Health and Social Care Board Belfast

Brown O (2016) Personal communication. Public Health Agency, Belfast

Cabinet Office & Northern Ireland Office (2013) Devolution settlement: Northern Ireland. Available via https://www.gov.uk/guidance/devolution-settlement-northern-ireland. Accessed 23 June 2016

Chartered Society of Physiotherapy (2016) New legislation on independent prescribing comes into effect on 1 June. Available via http://www.csp.org.uk/news/2015/05/12/new-legislation-independent-prescribing-comes-effect-1-june. Accessed 12 June 2017

Department of Health (2003) Supplementary prescribing by nurses and pharmacists with the NHS in England a guide for implementation [Archived]. Available via http://webarchive.nationalarchives.gov.uk/20130107105354/http://www.dh.gov.uk/en/Publicationsandstatistics/Publications/PublicationsPolicyAndGuidance/DH_4009717. Accessed 15 June 2016

Department of Health (2004) Outline curriculum for training programmes to prepare allied health professionals as supplementary prescribers. Available via http://webarchive.nationalarchives.gov.uk/20130107105354/http:/dh.gov.uk/en/publicationsandstatistics/publications/publicationspolicyandguidance/dh_4089002. Accessed 12 June 2017

Department of Health (2005a) Supplementary prescribing by nurses, pharmacists, chiropodists/podiatrists, physiotherapists and radiographers within the NHS in England. A guide for implementation. Updated May 2005. Department of Health, London

Department of Health (2005b) Supplementary prescribing by nurses, pharmacists, chiropodists/podiatrists, physiotherapists and radiographers within the NHS in England. A guide for implementation. Updated May 2005. Department of Health, London

Department of Health (2006) Improving patients' access to medicines: a guide to implementing nurse and pharmacist independent prescribing within the NHS in England. Available via http://webarchive.nationalarchives.gov.uk/20130107105354/http:/www.dh.gov.uk/prod_consum_dh/groups/dh_digitalassets/@dh/@en/documents/digitalasset/dh_4133747.pdf . Accessed 12 June 2017

Department of Health, Northern Ireland (2016a) Prescribing by non-medical healthcare professionals. Three types of non-medical prescribing.

Independent prescribing. Available via https://www.health-ni.gov.uk/articles/pharmaceutical-non-medical-prescribing. Accessed 9 June 2016

Department of Health, Northern Ireland, (2016b). Health and wellbeing 2026 – delivering together. Available via https://www.health-ni.gov.uk/publications/health-and-wellbeing-2026-delivering-together. Accessed 12 June 2017

Department of Health, Social Services and Public Safety (2004) Supplementary prescribing by nurses and pharmacists within the HPSS in Northern Ireland: a guide for implementation. Department of Health, Social Services and Public Safety, Belfast

Department of Health, Social Services and Public Safety (2006) Improving patients' access to medicines: a guide to implementing nurse and pharmacist independent prescribing within the HPSS in Northern Ireland. Department of Health, Social Services and Public Safety, Belfast

Department of Health, Social Services and Public Safety (2008a) Press release: prescriptions from your high street opticians. Optometrists to get independent prescribing powers. Available via www.publichealthagency.org/sites/default/.../Prescriptions%20press%20release_0.pdf. Accessed 12 June 2017

Department of Health, Social Services and Public Safety (2008b) Prescribing of controlled drugs by nurse independent prescribers. Mawhinney M, McLernon A. 22 May 2008. Available via https://www.health-ni.gov.uk/publications/advice-non-medical-prescribers. Accessed 15 June 2016

Department of Health, Social Services and Public Safety (2010) Review of development needs for pharmaceutical staff in hospital practice. Available via https://www.health-ni.gov.uk/publications/review-development-needs-pharmaceutical-staff-hospital-practice. Accessed 20 Oct 2016

Department of Health, Social Services and Public Safety (2011) Transforming your care: a review of health and social care in Northern Ireland. Available via https://www.health-ni.gov.uk/topics/health-policy/transforming-your-care. Accessed 22 Oct 2016

Department of Health, Social Services and Public Safety (2012a) The misuse of drugs (amendment) regulations (Northern Ireland) 2012. Morrow M, McLernon A. 30 Mar 2012. Available via https://www.health-ni.gov.uk/publications/controlled-drugs-misuse-drugs-regulations--amendments. Accessed 15 June 2016

Department of Health, Social Services and Public Safety (2012b) Developing eyecare partnerships: improving the commissioning and provision of eyecare services in Northern Ireland. Available via http://www.hscbusiness.hscni.net/pdf/DEVELOPING_EYECARE_PARTNERSHIPS_2012(1).pdf. Accessed 29 Aug 2016

Department of Health, Social Services and Public Safety (2015a) Non-medical prescribing: changes in legislation regarding mixing of medicines and prescribing unlicensed medicines. Bradley M, Morrow N. 4 Feb 2010. Available via https://www.health-ni.gov.uk/publications/advice-non-medical-prescribers. Accessed 15 June 2016

Department of Health, Social Services and Public Safety (2015b) Independent prescribing by physiotherapists and podiatrists or chiropodists. Timoney M, Winning H. 9 Jan 2015. Available via https://www.health-ni.gov.uk/publications/advice-independent-prescribing-by-physiotherapists-and-podiatrists. Accessed 15 June 2016

General Optical Council (2016) Search the register. Available via https://www.optical.org/en/utilities/online-registers.cfm. Accessed 8 June 2016

General Pharmaceutical Council (2016) Pharmacist independent prescribing programme—learning outcomes and indicative content. Available via https://www.pharmacyregulation.org/education/pharmacist-independent-prescriber. Accessed 21 Dec 2016

Health and Social Care Board (2016) Southern primary eyecare assessment and referral service (SPEARS) evaluation report. Available via http://www.hscbusiness.hscni.net/pdf/SPEARS_Evaluation_Report_March_2016.pdf. Accessed 29 Aug 2016

Mawhinney M (2016) Head of medicines regulatory group. Personal communication. Department of Health, Northern Ireland.

McClelland J (2016) Optometrist prescribing in Northern Ireland. Personal communication. Ulster University, Northern Ireland

McMullan M (2016) Optometrist prescribing in Northern Ireland. Personal communication. Health and Social Care Board Belfast, Northern Ireland

NICPLD (2016) Pharmacist supplementary and independent prescribing course. Personal communication. Northern Ireland

Northern Ireland Assembly (2016) Committee for health. Available via http://www.niassembly.gov.uk/assembly-business/committees/2016-2017/committee-for-health/. Accessed 12 June 2017

Northern Ireland Practice Education Council (NICPEC) (2014). A review into the impact and status of Nurse Prescribing in Northern Ireland. Available via http://www.nipec.n-i.nhs.uk/Image/SitePDFS/NursePrescribingFinal%2025%20April%202014.pdf. Accessed 12 June 2017

Northern Ireland Statistics and Research Agency (NISRA) (2016) The population of Northern Ireland. Available via https://www.nisra.gov.uk/statistics/population. Accessed 12 June 2017

Office for National Statistics (ONS) (2016) Population estimates, mid-year 2016. Available via https://www.ons.gov.uk/peoplepopulationandcommunity/populationandmigration/populationestimates/bulletins/annualmidyearpopulationestimates/latest. Accessed 12 June 2017

Royal Pharmaceutical Society of Great Britain (2003) Final report of pharmacist prescribing task group. Royal Pharmaceutical Society of Great Britain, London

Royal Pharmaceutical Society of Great Britain (2006a) Outline curriculum for training programmes to prepare pharmacist prescribers. Royal Pharmaceutical Society of Great Britain, London

Royal Pharmaceutical Society of Great Britain (2006b) Curriculum for the education and training of pharmacist supplementary prescribers to become independent prescribers. Royal Pharmaceutical Society of Great Britain, London

# Part II
# Non-medical Prescribing by Pharmacists and Allied Health Professionals

# Chapter 5
# Non-medical Prescribing by Pharmacists

Graham Brack

**Abstract**  At the time of writing (June 2016), there are 51,964 pharmacists registered with the General Pharmaceutical Council. Of these, 3761 are also registered as independent prescribers with an additional 949 who are supplementary prescribers (Personal communication from GPhC Registration Department 2016). There are two ways of viewing this. One might say that the introduction of pharmacist prescribing has generated an additional four and a half thousand prescribers, or one might ask why, 14 years after the opening of prescribing to pharmacists, only 3.76% of pharmacists have trained as prescribers, despite the advantages of doing so. This chapter will look at the history and development of pharmacist prescribing, the barriers, which have militated against faster uptake, and the potential that the profession has if these issues can be successfully addressed.

**Keywords**  Pharmacist • Autonomy • Repeat prescribing • Independent prescriber • Supplementary prescriber • Education • Dispensing • Minor ailments

---

G. Brack
Associate Lecturer, Plymouth University, Plymouth, UK
e-mail: postbox@grahambrack.com

© Springer International Publishing AG 2017
P.M. Franklin (ed.), *Non-medical Prescribing in the United Kingdom*,
DOI 10.1007/978-3-319-53324-7_5

## 5.1 Genesis

To many laypeople, the fact that non-medical prescribing was offered to nurses rather than to pharmacists, the profession specifically trained to have knowledge about the optimal use of drugs, seems perverse, but this was conditioned by the way in which nurse prescribing came about.

In 1986 the Department of Health and Social Security commissioned a report into the activities of district nurses and health visitors in people's homes. That report, commonly known after the name of the chairperson as the Cumberlege Report (DHSS 1986), was concerned primarily with making best use of community nursing resources. It drew particular attention to the difficulties faced by district nursing and health visitor teams in areas where their patients were drawn from the lists of a number of GP practices and made some suggestions for ameliorating the administrative burden that this multiplicity of links created, the notion being that less time spent on administration would mean more time available for direct patient care. One suggestion was that the need to return to a surgery so that a GP could provide a prescription for a patient under their care was an unnecessary burden given that in many cases the items required were wound dressings and topical applications that could be regarded as safe—and were commonly not subject to restrictions on supply under the Medicines Act 1968, so that patients could have purchased them themselves anyway. The report therefore proposed that a limited list of items could be drafted which nurses and health visitors would be able to prescribe.

While this may appear a self-evident and appropriate response now, it ought to be noted that the proposal did not meet with universal approbation when it was made. A letter to the Journal of the Royal College of General Practitioners (Holmes et al. 1985) does not take issue with the idea that nurses can be involved in some clinical decisions, including the prescription of certain medications and dressings, when properly supervised, and with clear lines of responsibility. However, the tone of this comment is not one suggesting autonomy in practice. The correspondents also noted that there was no evidence presented to back up some of the recommendations and were critical of the apparent endorsement of the Royal College of Nursing view that as a matter of professional principle, nurses should not be subject to control and direction by doctors over their professional work. This again suggests some disagreement about the principle of autonomous prescribing by nurses.

It is instructive to note that there was less controversy then about prescribing by pharmacists, simply because the matter was rarely discussed at all. As a young and newly qualified pharmacist in 1979, my first job was as a ward pharmacist on the chest, paediatric and gynaecology wards of a local hospital group. Ward pharmacy was a relatively new concept—it had not, for example, been mentioned during our university training—but the idea of placing pharmacists within wards was being well received. Our role was to answer questions raised by medical and nursing staff and to advise generally on the better use of medicines. Typically most of our contact was with the junior hospital doctors, who were mostly people of our own age and a similar level of experience, so that our advice could be considered peer support, but as ward pharmacists became embedded and joined ward rounds, it became more common to interact with registrars and consultants. This led to general acceptance of the principle that hospital pharmacists could amend prescriptions written by doctors. Initially this centred on errors or infelicities in prescribing such as brands not stocked in that hospital, but as time progressed, it came to include changing brands to generic alternatives except where hospital policy did not permit it. None of these powers were proposed for their community colleagues as yet, and the World Health Organization paper (WHO 1994) explained why this should be so. Hospital pharmacists generally had easy access to medical notes, which was denied to community pharmacists and commonly had regular face-to-face contact with the prescribers, which permitted them to exercise a role in education and medicines management. This document still drew a distinction between the pharmacist role and prescribing, but increasingly the gap was being narrowed. It did not matter that the term *pharmacist prescriber* was not used, because the effect of the ward pharmacist's activities was very similar.

Thus there was little impetus to promote pharmacist prescribing at the time of the Cumberlege Report (1986). In hospital pharmacy it was felt to be unnecessary because pharmacists already influenced and adjusted prescribing decisions, and in community practice the lack of access to key patient information was thought to preclude it.

There was also a view that there might be safety risks in allowing pharmacists to prescribe. This was not because they lacked knowledge but resulted from their position as the safety backstops reviewing doctors' prescriptions. It was argued that if pharmacists were prescribers, that valuable function would be missing.

The government established a further advisory group to examine the proposal for nurse prescribing under the chairmanship of Dr June Crown. It is important for our purposes here to note that the remit of the group only covered nurse prescribing. There was no interest in advancing pharmacist prescribing, and so neither the Crown Report (Department of Health 1989) itself nor the legislation permitting nurse prescribing that issued from it (Medicinal Products: Prescription by Nurses Act 1992) made mention of the possibility. In the first edition of the Pharmaceutical Journal of the 2000s, Keith Farrar was asked to "think the unthinkable" and offered what has proved to be a highly prescient view of hospital pharmacy in the new millennium, but nowhere does he mention pharmacist prescribing (Farrar 2000). However, within the community there was already some pressure for extension of prescribing powers.

It had not escaped the notice of pharmacists that some of the arguments used to advance nurse prescribing were equally valid for pharmacists; in particular, that extending prescribing to them would ease the administrative burden on hard-pressed general practitioners and would encourage the acceptance of pharmacists as part of the wider primary care team. There had been some pilot projects that appeared to support this such as one in Tayside which became an exemplar for repeat dispensing services but had been devised to reduce the workload of repeat prescribing (Dowell et al. 1998). Moreover, there was clear evidence that pharmacist involvement in prescribing improved quality of care (Hanlon et al. 1996) and a number of community medicines supply schemes had been successfully operated by pharmacists using Patient Group Directions introduced under Health Services Circular 2000/026 in the wake of the initial Crown Report.

A second Crown Report on the advisability of extending prescribing to professions other than nursing was commissioned by the Department of Health and was delivered in 1999 (Department of Health 1999). This report stated that "the current arrangements fail to make the fullest use of the skills of many professionals" (p. 27) and recommended that authority to prescribe should be extended beyond currently authorised prescribers to include new groups of healthcare professionals in specific therapeutic areas with expertise in these areas. In the light of the differences in training of doctors, nurses and pharmacists in relation to preparing a diagnosis, the report recommended a distinction between independent prescribers, who would be responsible for the initial assessment of the patient and devising the treatment plan, and dependent prescribers, who would be able to prescribe certain medicines for patients whose condition had been diagnosed by an independent prescriber when working within an agreed treatment plan ("supplementary prescriber" as being a more appropriate description of the professional relationship soon replaced the term "dependent prescriber"). The publication of this report was welcomed by the Pharmaceutical Journal in a leader article just 11 weeks after that quoted earlier (Pharmaceutical Journal 2000, p. 423). The author noted that "This is, indeed, welcome news for the profession and goes some way to filling the gaping void created by the continuing absence of the long-awaited community pharmacy strategy" and that "No opportunity should be missed to remind Ministers that a prescribing role, and with it full membership of the health care team, is what pharmacy wants".

The role offered under the second Crown Report was the dependent or supplementary role and therefore did not bring the full independence that some might have hoped for, but the Pharmaceutical Journal was content for the moment. The editorial opined that:

> Becoming dependent prescribers, able to make amendments to repeat prescriptions, would allow the medicines management proposals being developed for pharmacy by the PSNC to be implemented in full. Pharmacists would be able to make changes which were in the interests of patients' health, offering the patients a more tailored and responsive service, rather than simply referring them back to the initial prescriber every time. This is in line with the Government's desire for a modernised National Health Service. (Pharmaceutical Journal 2000, p. 423).

## 5.2   Implementation and Its Challenges

In 2003, the provisions of the Health and Social Care Act 2001 which permitted pharmacists to become supplementary prescribers came into effect, followed in 2006 by *The National Health Service (Miscellaneous Amendments Relating to Independent Prescribing) Regulations 2006* which allowed them to become independent prescribers. Before courses could be offered, it was necessary for universities to apply for accreditation for their courses from the Royal Pharmaceutical Society of Great Britain (RPSGB), which, until it ceded authority to the new General Pharmaceutical Council in 2010, was responsible for assuring standards of education. (There is a separate Pharmaceutical Society of Northern Ireland, which retains a similar responsibility as the registration authority for pharmacy in that country.)

It was decided at an early stage that a restriction similar to that for nurses was necessary to ensure that pharmacists had a certain level of experience before attempting a prescribing course, and candidates must therefore have completed 2 years in practice after the end of their preregistration year. It was further stipulated that these 2 years must be completed in a role which is *patient-orientated* so that pharmacists who work primarily in educational or industrial practice would not qualify.

In the case of nurses, it was expected that they would already possess some examination and consultation skills, so their prescribing training contained some emphasis on pharmacology. By contrast, pharmacists will have had a sound grounding in pharmacology during their undergraduate training but—at that time—may not have been trained in consultation and examination. RPSGB therefore gave notice that as university accreditations fell due for renewal, they would expect to see amendments to their undergraduate syllabi to incorporate more education in these skills. It was widely accepted that even pharmacists who chose not to become prescribers would benefit from these changes, as pharmaceutical practice was increasingly concerned with the management of minor ailments and the triage role that came from being readily accessible healthcare professionals.

With the introduction of independent prescribing, very few pharmacists have not preferred to take the independent prescribing course, and those who have qualified as supplementary prescribers have been able to undertake a conversion course provided that they have practised as supplementary prescribers in the 2 years before conversion and can produce evidence of satisfactory practice in this respect. Courses for the independent prescribing qualification usually last for a minimum of 6 months and are run on a blended learning part-time basis with face-to-face teaching days and some self-directed study. The programmes involve 26 days of teaching and learning activity and completion of at least 12 days of learning in a practice environment being mentored by a designated medical practitioner such as a general practitioner. The required clinical and diagnostics skills are taught as part of the course, and the designated medical practitioner will reinforce these in practice. A list of higher education institutions which, at the date of publishing, offer the pharmacist prescribing courses appears in Table 5.1.

There have been three additional requirements, which may have acted as a deterrent to some pharmacists, particularly in community practice. The candidate is required to have identified an area of clinical practice in which to develop their prescribing skills and have up-to-date clinical, pharmacological, and pharmaceutical knowledge relevant to their intended area of prescribing practice. This has been relatively easy for those employed in hospitals but is not so straightforward in community practice where specialisation is harder to achieve.

This was accentuated by a decision that pharmacists should also have identified a budget against which their prescribing would be charged. This led to a chicken-and-egg problem for some; having identified an area in which their expertise could be of value, they had to secure a budget for their work, but the budget was unlikely to be forthcoming unless they could demonstrate a track record of achievement. Experience has shown that even after qualification, this continues to be an issue for some pharmacists, whose projected service has not come into effect or has been terminated due to the financial difficulties that commissioners have faced.

A second difficulty is found in the separation of the prescribing and dispensing roles. One of the valued features of pharmacist practice is that the dispenser acts as a safety check

**Table 5.1** Higher education institutions accredited to provide pharmacist prescribing programmes. Updated 16th June 2017

| Name | Offering pharmacy degree (P = provisional) | Independent prescribing course | Conversion from supplementary to independent |
|---|---|---|---|
| Anglia Ruskin | | ✓ | |
| Aston University | ✓ | ✓ | |
| Bangor University | | ✓ | |
| University of Bath | ✓ | ✓ | |
| University of Belfast | | ✓ | |
| University of Birmingham | P | ✓ | |
| University of Bolton | | ✓ | |
| University of Bradford | ✓ | ✓ | |
| University of Brighton | ✓ | ✓ | |
| Cardiff University | ✓ | ✓ | |
| University of Central Lancashire | ✓ | ✓ | |
| University of Chester | | ✓ | |
| University of Coventry | | ✓ | |
| University of Cumbria | | ✓ | |
| De Montfort University | ✓ | ✓ | ✓ |
| University of Derby | | ✓ | |
| Durham University | P | | |
| University of East Anglia | ✓ | ✓ | |
| Edge Hill University | | ✓ | |
| Glyndŵr University | | ✓ | |
| University of Hertfordshire | ✓ | ✓ | |

(continued)

**Table 5.1** (continued)

| Name | Offering pharmacy degree (P = provisional) | Independent prescribing course | Conversion from supplementary to independent |
|---|---|---|---|
| University of Huddersfield | ✓ | | |
| University of Hull | | ✓ | |
| Keele University | ✓ | ✓ | |
| King's College London | ✓ | ✓ | |
| Kingston University London | ✓ | | |
| University of Leeds | | ✓ | ✓ |
| University of Lincoln | P | ✓ | |
| Liverpool John Moores University | ✓ | ✓ | |
| London South Bank University | | ✓ | |
| University College London | ✓ | | |
| University of Manchester | ✓ | ✓ | |
| Medway School of Pharmacy | ✓ | ✓ | |
| University of Nottingham | ✓ | | |
| University of Portsmouth | ✓ | ✓ | |
| University of Reading | | ✓ | ✓ |
| Robert Gordon University | | ✓ | |
| University of Salford | | ✓ | |
| Sheffield Halham University | | ✓ | |

**Table 5.1** (continued)

| Name | Offering pharmacy degree (P = provisional) | Independent prescribing course | Conversion from supplementary to independent |
|---|---|---|---|
| University of South Wales (formerly University of Glamorgan and University of Wales) | | ✓ | |
| University of Strathclyde | | ✓ | ✓ |
| University of Suffolk (formally University Campus Suffolk) | | ✓ | |
| University of Sunderland | | ✓ | |
| Swansea University | | ✓ | |
| University of West of England | | ✓ | |
| University of Wolverhampton | | ✓ | |
| University of Worcester | | ✓ | |
| University of York | | ✓ | |

Source: General Pharmaceutical Council website (www.pharmacyregulation.org) updated 16th June 2017

on the prescriber's prescriptions, and it would not be in the interests of the patient to allow this check to be abolished by having the prescriber and the dispenser being the same person. Accordingly, the rule has been adopted that a pharmacist prescriber should not dispense their own prescriptions except in cases of emergency. This is workable when a pharmacist works in a large pharmacy with two pharmacists, but the majority of community pharmacists do not have this luxury.

As a result, most prescribing by community pharmacists takes place in settings outside their pharmacy on a sessional basis. This still has value, but it is often not what was envisaged when services were proposed. It may also confuse clinical governance and lines of accountability; the wise prescribing pharmacist will ensure at the outset that all concerned are very clear about the governance and insurance arrangements that have been made to cover his or her practice.

The third difficulty frequently expressed by community staff is the requirement for a designated medical practitioner to oversee their clinical study days and act as mentor. In acute and partnership trusts, this role may well be fulfilled by a doctor within the team that will benefit from the new prescriber. In the community the demands of supervising GP registrars and medical students mean that GPs are reluctant to commit themselves to additional mentoring, especially since it is unfunded.

In a survey of pharmacist independent prescribing undertaken for Public Health Wales (Hinchliffe 2015), Anne Hinchliffe noted that while about one in eight pharmacist independent prescribers works in community pharmacy across the United Kingdom, there were only two in Wales. She further identified factors that promoted and hindered the development of the prescribing pharmacist role (Table 5.2):

## 5.3   Minor Ailments Schemes

The NHS community pharmacy contractual framework in England defines three levels of service (PSNC 2016). All NHS pharmacies must provide the essential services, which are seven in number:

**Table 5.2** Factors influencing the implementation of pharmacist prescribing

| Facilitators | Barriers |
|---|---|
| Support from colleagues | Lack of support and awareness from other healthcare professionals |
| Having appropriate knowledge and experience | Difficulty assessing patients |
| Dedicated time | Lack of time |
| Funding | Lack of funding |
| Good communication | Limited opportunities |
| A good relationship with the patient's doctor | The need for a second pharmacist to clinically check the prescription before dispensing |
| Access to shared records | Inadequate access to medical records |

Source: Hinchliffe A, Pharmacist independent prescribing—a review of the evidence, Public Health Wales, 2015

- Dispensing appliances
- Dispensing medicines
- Disposal of unwanted medicines
- Public health (promotion of healthy lifestyles)
- Repeat dispensing
- Signposting
- Support for self-care

There are also advanced services, which are commissioned by NHS England on a national basis and which can be provided by any pharmacy that meets the accreditation standards for each service. These include the new medicines service and medicine use reviews.

In addition, local health economies may commission enhanced services, which are specified locally and which must be funded locally too. One of the most popular of these services has been a minor ailments service. These are also found in the devolved nations.

A minor ailments service is designed to allow patients to obtain rapid treatment for specified conditions from a pharmacy without the need for a doctor's appointment. Since these conditions are usually common, the service can produce a considerable reduction in GP and emergency department workload, and since the fees offered to pharmacists are usually lower than any other disposition, there may be a cost saving too.

Since the scope of each service is locally determined, the conditions, which may be treated, vary from area to area, but to give one example, the minor ailments scheme in Cornwall allows treatment of urinary tract infections in women, impetigo limited to one or two areas, conjunctivitis, nappy rash and oral thrush using specified products. The mode of supply is using Patient Group Directions which allow supply to patients who meet diagnostic criteria and do not possess any excluding features. In effect, a Patient Group Direction is rather like a prescription with the patient's name left off, which is then completed by the healthcare professional permitted by the Patient Group Direction to do so. Having diagnosed the condition and made a supply, the pharmacist reports the interaction to the patient's GP for inclusion in their medical history and claims reimbursement for the medicines used, plus an agreed fee, from the local NHS.

Evaluations of these schemes have been extremely positive. Pumtong and colleagues (Pumtong et al. 2011) evaluated a scheme in Nottingham and concluded "The majority of stakeholders perceived benefits of the scheme for both patients and health care professionals. The level of patient satisfaction with the scheme was high, particularly in terms of ease of access and convenience".

Baqir and colleagues (Baqir et al. 2011) asked whether such schemes do indeed reduce demand on GP services and concluded that they do. A scheme in three primary care trusts was estimated to save around £6739 per month. Evaluations of similar schemes in Scotland (Wagner et al. 2011), Wales and Northern Ireland (McCarthy et al. 2015) produced a consistent level of satisfaction and outcomes.

However, it can be argued that it is the very success of these minor ailments schemes, and similar schemes for the provision of smoking cessation products and emergency hormonal contraception, that have acted as a brake upon pharmacist prescribing.

As part of the review into the supply of medicines, the Crown Report (Department of Health 1999) had expressed dissatisfaction with the use of group protocols, local forerunners of Patient Group Directions, which had been developed in some hospitals but which, in the committee's view, were not sufficiently subject to good governance practice. The committee expressed a strong preference for individualised care (though noting that even after an expansion of prescribing rights, there might remain some need for group prescribing arrangements). This suggested that, while an expansion in the use of Patient Group Directions might be needed until healthcare professionals were trained as prescribers, in time many of them would fall into disuse as individualised care by practitioners taking full responsibility for their prescribing became more numerous. This has not happened.

Instead, while prescribing has been opened up to many health professions, the use of Patient Group Directions has continued to grow, and it is arguable that employers have not felt the need to put staff forward for prescribing training so long as Patient Group Directions remain available.

Nowhere has this been more marked than in pharmacy, where minor ailments schemes depend on Patient Group Directions and are not open to pharmacist prescribers as such. As a result, pharmacists like myself have found ourselves providing medicines under Patient Group Directions that we might have prescribed in other circumstances while finding it hard to have services that rely on prescribing commissioned.

## 5.4  Pharmacists in GP Practices

In 2015 NHS England announced a pilot worth £31m under which 470 pharmacists would work in around 700 GP practices over 3 years providing additional clinical support. Such was the enthusiasm for this project that within a few months a further £112m had been committed to expand the number to 1500 or more (Sukkar 2016).

The roles that these pharmacists will occupy has not yet been clearly defined, except that they will be expected to be undertaking clinical rather than administrative tasks, but it is reasonable to suppose that the appetite of GPs for the help of pharmacists will be a major determinant, and one such GP provided a bullish commentary of the prospects for this programme (Parkin 2016).

Dr Parkin's analysis is trenchant and challenging:

> This scheme is undervaluing the skills pharmacists have to offer in general practice. It should have an aim of creating pharmacist advanced clinical practitioners operating independently to diagnose, investigate, treat and refer patients as appropriate. (Via http://www.pharmaceutical-journal.com/opinion/correspondence/pharmacy-must-grasp-new-clinical-opportunities-with-both-hands/20200979.article; Accessed 13 June 2017).

One issue that remains to be worked through is the tension between access and good planning. It is often said—not least by pharmacy's professional organisations—that one of the great advantages of community pharmacy is its ready accessibility. Pharmacies are situated on high streets and do not operate appointment systems. However, one of the lessons of the introduction of advanced services into the community pharmacy contract is that these are very difficult to provide adequately on a walk-in basis, and therefore pharmacies have increasingly adopted booking systems for them in order to balance supply and demand. There has been concern that when plans are made to divert patients from GPs to pharmacies, very often it is the unplanned or emergency work that is easiest to move. This eases GP workload, but it creates major problems for pharmacies, which find that they have more volatile workflows and that demand for prescribing services detracts from the efficient dispensing service that has long been their major role. For this reason many pharmacist prescribers are keen to concentrate on the management of long-term conditions, where a relationship can be established with a patient and care provided on a diarized basis.

The prospects for pharmacist advanced clinical practitioners would be considerably enhanced if there were a cadre of pharmacist prescribers ready to take independent responsibility for the management of long-term conditions, which make up so large a part of GP workload. Pharmacist prescribing may have had a stuttering start, but its future could be very bright indeed, to the benefit of patients and professionals alike.

**DHSSPNI**
Cathy Harrison, Senior Principal Pharmaceutical Officer, Department of Health, Castle Buildings, Stormont. Belfast BT43SQ

Mary Frances McManus, Nursing Officer, Department of Health, Castle Buildings, Stormont. Belfast BT43SQ

Hazel Winning, AHP Lead officer, Department of Health, Castle Buildings, Stormont. Belfast BT43SQ

**Health and Social Care Board**
Chris Blayney, Pharmacy Adviser, Health and Social Care Board, Belfast

Glynis Boyd-McMurtry, Medicines Management Co-ordinator, Health and Social Care Board, Belfast

Margaret McMullan, Clinical Optometric Adviser, Health and Social Care Board, Belfast

**Hospital Trusts**
The following pharmacists supplied up-to-date figures for the number of prescribing pharmacists working across the five hospital trusts in Northern Ireland:

Jayne Agnew, Clinical Pharmacy Manager, Southern Health and Social Care Trust

Alison Campbell, Clinical Pharmacy Development Lead. South Eastern Health and Social Care Trust

Paula Crawford, Lead Clinical Pharmacist, Musgrave Park Hospital, Belfast Health and Social Care Trust

Dianne Gill, Deputy Head Pharmacy and Medicines Management, Northern Health and Social Care Trust

Brendan Moore, Clinical Pharmacy Manager, Western Health and Social Care Trust

Dr Roisin O'Hare, Clinical pharmacist, Queen's University Belfast

**NICPLD, Queen's University Belfast**
Prof. C.G. Adair, Director, NICPLD
Laura O'Loan, Assistant Director, NICPLD

**Public Health Agency**
Oriel Brown, Nurse Consultant: Service Development, Service Improvement, Public Health Agency

Michelle Tennyson, Assistant Director Allied Health Professions and Personal and Public Involvement, Public Health Agency

**Ulster University**
Kerry Clarke. Lecturer in Podiatry, School of Health Sciences, Ulster University

Dr Julie McClelland. Lecturer in Optometry, School of Biomedical Sciences, Ulster University

# References

Baqir W, Learoyd T, Sim A, Todd A (2011) Cost analysis of a community pharmacy 'minor ailment scheme' across three primary care trusts in the North East of England. J Public Health 33(4):551–555

Department of Health (1989) Report of the advisory group on nurse prescribing (Crown Report). The Stationery Office, London

Department of Health (1999) Review of prescribing, supply and administration of medicines. Final report. Stationery Office, London

Department of Health and Social Security (1986) Neighbourhood nurs-
    ing—a focus for care (The Cumberlege Report). HMSO, London

Dowell J, Cruikshank J, Bain J et al (1998) Repeat dispensing by commu-
    nity pharmacists: advantages for patients and practitioners. Br J Gen
    Pract 48:1858–1859

Farrar K (2000) Hospital pharmacy: thinking the unthinkable. Pharm
    J Available via http://www.pharmaceutical-journal.com/in-depth/%20
    perspective-article/hospital-pharmacy-thinking-the-unthink-%20
    able/20000004.article. Accessed 13 June 2017

Hanlon JT, Samsa GP, Lewis IK, Landsman PB (1996) A randomised con-
    trolled trial of a clinical pharmacist intervention to improve inappropri-
    ate prescribing in elderly outpatients with polypharmacy. Am J Med
    100:428–437

Hinchliffe A (2015) Pharmacist independent prescribing—a review of the
    evidence. Public Health Wales

Holmes W, Armstrong R, Oliver P (1985) The Cumberlege Report—another
    view. J R Coll Gen Pract 36(291):474–475

McCarthy A, O'Nolan G, Long J (2015) *Minor ailments schemes: an over-
    view of experience up to 2015*, for the Health Research Board, for a
    review of schemes and evaluations in a number of countries. Available
    via    http://www.hrb.ie/uploads/tx_hrbpublications/Minor_ailments_
    schemes_an_overview_of_experience_up_to_2015_01.pdf.    Accessed
    13 June 2017

Medicinal Products: Prescription by Nurses Act (1992) Available via http://
    www.uklaws.org/statutory/instruments_13/doc13024.htm. Accessed 21
    Dec 2016

Parkin T (2016) Pharmacy must grasp new clinical opportunities with both
    hands. Clin Pharmacist 8(5). doi: 10.1211/CP.2016.20200979

Pharmaceutical Journal Editorial (2000) Pharmacist prescribing—one step
    closer. Pharm J 264(7088):p423

PSNC    (2016)    Available    via    http://psnc.org.uk/contract-it/the-phar-
    macy-%20contract/. Accessed 13 June 2017

Pumtong S, Boardman HF, Anderson CW (2011) A multi-method evalua-
    tion of the pharmacy first minor ailments scheme. Int J Clin Pharm
    33(3):573–581

Sukkar E (2016) GP surgeries could employ an extra 1500 pharmacists with
    £112m investment. Pharm J 296(7888). doi: 10.1211/PJ.2016.20201055

Wagner A, Noyce PR, Ashcroft DM (2011) Changing patient consultation
    patterns in primary care: an investigation of uptake of the minor ail-
    ments Service in Scotland. Health Policy 99(1):44–51

WHO (1994) The role of the pharmacist in the health care system. Available via
    http://apps.who.int/medicinedocs/en/d/Jh2995e/. Accessed 21 Dec 2016

# Chapter 6
# Prescribing by Designated Allied Health Professionals: The AHP Experience

Alan Borthwick, Tim Kilmartin, Nicky Wilson, and Christina Freeman

**Abstract** To date, only three allied health professions are approved as independent prescribers, notably physiotherapy, podiatry and therapeutic radiography, with diagnostic radiography and dietetics approved as supplementary prescribers. This chapter provides an insight into recent experiences of the enactment and implementation of independent prescribing for these professions and highlights the advantages, obstacles and potential future developments in allied health prescribing.

**Keywords** Allied health professions • Independent prescribing • Physiotherapy • Podiatry • Radiography

A. Borthwick (✉)
Centre for Innovation and Leadership in Health Sciences, University of Southampton, Building 45, Highfield, Southampton SO17 1BJ, UK
e-mail: ab12@soton.ac.uk

T. Kilmartin
Ilkeston Community Hospital, Derbyshire Community Health Services, NHS Foundation Trust, Derbyshire, UK

N. Wilson
King's College, London, UK

C. Freeman
Society and College of Radiographers, London, UK

© Springer International Publishing AG 2017      113
P.M. Franklin (ed.), *Non-medical Prescribing in the United Kingdom*,
DOI 10.1007/978-3-319-53324-7_6

## 6.1   Introduction

It would be all too easy to view the acquisition of prescribing
rights by the allied health professions as a smooth and linear
process, but to do so would fail to capture the complexity
involved or to appreciate the underlying drivers for such change.
Indeed, the move towards allied health prescribing largely
reflects an evolving health policy agenda designed to address
both workforce and demographic concerns (Borthwick 2008).
Equally, it is important to acknowledge the relevance of professional power relationships in determining role boundaries
(Freidson 1988; Larkin 1988, 1993; Freidson 2001; Saks 2013,
2014). In order to make sense of the gradual shift in prescribing
roles across the various allied health professions, it is helpful to
acknowledge the underlying influences that have shaped the
change. Whilst each allied health profession has a unique story,
they share a common narrative informed by the workforce redesign agenda aimed at ensuring a sustainable healthcare system
responsive to growing and changing patient need (Davies 2003;
Duckett 2005). Although the forces driving change are common
to the allied health professions, their experience of prescribing
varies. Some do not yet have any form of prescribing rights and
may not even intend to pursue them, whilst others enjoy a wide
range of access mechanisms allowing practitioners of varying
levels and clinical experience to supply, sell, administer and
prescribe medicines.

## 6.2   The Allied Health Professions

At present, only three allied health professions enjoy 'independent' prescriber status: physiotherapy, podiatry and therapeutic
radiography. They may also act as supplementary prescribers, as
may diagnostic radiographers and dieticians. Optometrists and

pharmacists have independent prescribing responsibilities, although, curiously, they are not generally regarded as 'allied health professions'. Regulated separately, they have a distinctly different sociohistorical context and have not, as a result, been included in the group of professions known today as 'allied health' (Larkin 1983, 1988, 2002). Indeed, the problematic progress of allied health prescribing stems from the professions' earlier status as 'auxiliary to medicine', evolving first to 'supplementary to medicine', before becoming 'allied to medicine' (or even, most recently, 'allied to each other'(Boyce 2006)), reflecting a gradual shift from subordinate and supportive roles to independent professional status in a hierarchical health division of labour (Larkin 1988, 1993, 1995, 2002; Saks 2014). It is against this background that the gradual acquisition of prescribing rights by the allied health professions must be considered, as they have had to work hard to justify their claims to an often sceptical audience (Borthwick et al. 2010; Borthwick 2012, 2013). Each of these professions shares a similar experience in having to construct a detailed and robust case for submission, with a common set of hurdles to clear before approval is granted. The need to construct formal professional practice guidance documents, relevant outline curricular frameworks to guide education and training, impact assessments, equality analyses and consultation summaries, not to mention the laborious and time-consuming processes of stakeholder consultations and public consultations, illustrates the commitment, skills and perseverance required.

But who exactly are the 'allied health professions', and which of them are able to access, supply, administer and prescribe medicines? The answer is more complicated than it might at first appear. At present, the Health and Care Professions Council registers 16 professions, not all of whom refer to themselves as 'allied health professions'. Whilst there are no clear criteria describing an *allied health* profession, it is a term which is broadly applied to those professions previously registered as 'supplementary to medicine' under the Act of Parliament bearing that name (*Professions Supplementary to Medicine Act 1960*). Today, the Allied Health Professions Federation (a leadership organisation giving a collective voice to the allied health professions) has 12 member organisations, of which only nine presently enjoy any form of rights to access restricted medicines. Of these, only four have been granted actual prescribing rights and only three (or, to be exact, two and half of one) full independent prescribing rights. Early in 2016, *the Commission on Human Medicines* announced it would support the submission for independent prescribing by therapeutic radiographers, but not by diagnostic radiographers, effectively establishing a legal distinction between the two arms of that profession.

## 6.3   Allied Health Independent Prescribing: Physiotherapy, Podiatry and Therapeutic Radiography

All three professions are relative newcomers to independent prescribing, with legislation coming into effect in August 2013 for podiatry and physiotherapy and 2016 for therapeutic radiography. Thus, only physiotherapists and podiatrists have had actual experience of the processes involved, from education and training through to independent prescribing practice. At the time of writing, the most recent figures available from the HCPC indicate that there are 303 physiotherapist and 151 podiatrist independent prescribers, from a register of 48,000 and 13,000, respectively. In other words, a relatively small proportion of these professions has, to date (June 2016), undertaken the training and qualified (and registered) as independent prescribers. In part this may be because the outline curriculum framework documents require all applicants to the independent prescribing programmes to have been qualified and practising as podiatrists or physiotherapists for at least 3 years and to have the approval of their employers in order to proceed (AHPF 2013a, b). Most are, therefore, already experienced practitioners in their given fields, and many have been accustomed to acquiring and using medicines relevant to their speciality field of practice by other means (such as supplementary prescribing, patient group directions or statutory exemption lists). Many will have been supplementary prescribers prior to becoming independent prescribers (physiotherapists, radiographers and podiatrists have been able to act as supplementary prescribers since 2005) (Department of Health 2005).

In the absence of access to research data from the formal evaluation of physiotherapist and podiatrist prescribing presently being undertaken by the universities of Brighton and Surrey (as part of the DH-commissioned study), this chapter reports the experiences to date of the authors of the chapter, which include a practising independent prescriber physiotherapist (a consultant physiotherapist), an independent prescriber podiatrist (a consultant podiatric surgeon), the professional officer of the Society and College of Radiographers and a former chairman of the College of Podiatry medicines committee; the latter two authors represented the allied health professions on the Department of Health Allied Health Professions Medicines Project Boards.

## 6.4 Podiatry and Physiotherapy: Current Issues

**Education and Training** The first notable challenge has been the generic, multi-professional form of education and training in prescribing. Early on in the planning of the submission to the Commission on Human Medicines (CHM) for physiotherapy and podiatry, it became clear that the viability of educational programmes could only be ensured if they were delivered alongside, and as part of, the broader prescribing education for nurses and pharmacists. Too few initial applicants would clearly make it difficult to justify separate programmes. In itself this brought the challenge of making the experience relevant to the clinical practice of podiatrists and physiotherapists. Use of a personal formulary, drawn from the nursing model, provided a means to ensure specific needs were catered for, and this enables practitioners to develop their skills within a specialist domain.

As a personal example from practice, within podiatric surgery, it was clear that the course work involved provided an opportunity to review key issues directly linked to actual surgical practice, including the management of osteomyelitis, the prophylaxis of infection and the prophylaxis of veno-thromboembolism. At present, these are areas where there is little consensus, and the opportunity to focus attention on exploring the evidence enabled the development of some specific guidelines for practice.

**The Designated Medical Practitioner (DMP) as Mentor**  In line with earlier templates for non-medical prescribing education and training programmes, both academic and practice elements are involved, and the practical prescribing components require the support of a mentor in practice—a 'designated medical practitioner' (DMP) willing to act as a mentor who will oversee and assess the prescribing activity of the trainee. It is very evident that this aspect of the education and training of allied health prescribers is vitally important and yet also potentially the biggest single obstacle to undertaking the programme. Finding a medical practitioner willing, interested or even available to mentor an AHP in training for 90 hours of clinical practice (the prescribed number of hours required) is likely to pose difficulties for those working in relative isolation, as many podiatrists do, for example.

At present the outline curricular framework documents require that mentors in practice—the 'designated medical practitioner'—must be medically qualified (AHPF 2013a). To date, some AHPs have even asked their professional body for a 'list' of DMPs to be circulated to those wishing to undertake the prescribing programme (needless to say, such a list does not exist). This has required some innovative strategies to persuade doctors to take part, including the use of incentives in one form or another. Often a quid pro quo arrangement has been necessary, in which the practitioner is able to offer some tangible benefit to the GP or physician involved. At one level, the mere fact that there is an opportunity to share the prescribing workload would seem enough of an incentive, but this alone cannot always be taken for granted.

Equally, it is tempting to imagine that it is simply a matter of time before sufficient numbers of independent prescriber AHPs are experienced enough to become DMPs and to assume that this would be a desirable longer-term outcome. The reality may be more complicated. At present, doctors may well be best suited to continue to act as DMPs, given their broader training and experience of multiple morbidities. The sheer complexity of the cases presenting in practice is a challenge, and the management of patients with long-term, multiple comorbidities may well complicate the picture for specialist AHP practitioners expert in a given field but less accustomed to managing across a wide breadth of disorders.

## 6.5  Independent Prescribing in Practice: Key Advantages

Once qualified and registered with the appropriate annotation, physiotherapist and podiatrist independent prescribers appear able to provide medicines to patients in a more timely manner than is afforded via other existing mechanisms and are able to do so appropriately, as was originally envisaged when allied health prescribing was first proposed in the Crown Report in 1999 (Department of Health 1999). Indeed, experience to date suggests that where the independent prescribing privilege is used regularly, it has effectively superseded the use of patient group directions

(PGDs) and other access mechanisms that might have been previously available to AHPs. For example, one practitioner working in an NHS trust for 22 years had amassed up to 20 PGDs to obtain the medicines necessary for practice (as a podiatric surgeon). After qualifying as an independent prescriber, however, he was able to prescribe anticoagulants for patients who had been placed in plaster of paris casts. This would not have been possible through the use of PGDs, as they do not authorise the practitioner to supply subcuticular low molecular weight heparin for administration by a district nurse. IP has also enabled podiatric surgeons to prescribe gabapentin for the management of poor pain control and to access new oral anticoagulants, which are preferable to the use of injectable forms that were available previously.

Nor is the positive experience of independent prescribing confined to NHS practice. Independent prescribing in the private sector, as envisaged in the Department of Health AHP Medicines Prescribing Project, would also seem to be proving a realistic and viable activity to some extent, at least in secondary care. Podiatric surgical practice in one private hospital, for example, has been enhanced by the advent of independent podiatric prescribing, enabling access to the required drugs without difficulty, thus avoiding the need to 'beg a favour' of medical colleagues busy with their own patients and uncertain about who would be responsible for any adverse outcomes, whilst ensuring minimal inconvenience to the patients.

## 6.6  Independent Prescribing in Practice: Disadvantages

Certain obstacles to practice have already arisen which give some indication of the limitations inherent in the existing processes. For example, the limited formulary of controlled drugs approved for physiotherapy and podiatry (those for therapeutic radiography are not yet approved by the Home Office) is proving a challenge, because of the lack of flexibility in finding alternatives to those drugs listed. Experience in physiotherapy practice, for example, has shown that the limitations imposed by a specified list can force the prescriber to resort to supplementary prescribing in order to obtain the appropriate drug. Another option would be to write a separate patient group direction (PGD) for the alternative CD not on the approved list, but this would be a laborious and time-consuming process and is unlikely to be a popular method.

Furthermore, although independent AHP prescribers have access to most drugs in the BNF, they are often constrained by local formularies that are shaped by financial considerations, which limit medicines. This may also influence prescribing activity, where specific budgetary lines determine who undertakes the prescribing. Experience suggests that acute Trusts may actively choose to limit prescribing due to financial constraints. In some instances, for example, a physiotherapist may wish to prescribe a non-steroidal anti-inflammatory medicine or a proton pump inhibitor but find they may be inhibited from doing so because the remit given to them is to refer the prescribing back to the patient's GP, so that the cost is transferred to the GP budget.

## 6.7  Radiography: Current Issues

**To Be or Not to Be? Diagnostic Radiography** Whilst the examples of physiotherapy and podiatry are largely relevant to AHP practice within both primary care and the private sector, radiography is a profession firmly rooted in secondary care. Following the decision of the Commission on Human Medicines (CHM) to grant independent prescribing rights to therapeutic, but not diagnostic radiography, a curious dichotomy has arisen, which has no precedent. Radiographers have had access to patient group directions since 2000, and been eligible for supplementary prescribing since 2005, but are now faced with a situation where only those involved with the delivery of medicines in cancer care (therapeutic radiographers) may do so independently. It is clear that this has important implications for practice across the profession.

Diagnostic radiographers play a key role in establishing a diagnosis from the use of imaging methods such as CT, MRI or PET scans, often involving the administration of contrast agents (all of which are prescription-only medicines) (Hogg and Hogg 2006; Hogg et al. 2007). Presently, it is difficult to operate this system using patient group directions (PGDs), although they are the only available mechanisms in such instances. Where radiologists are present, they are able to provide the necessary authority, but there is a shortage of qualified radiologists, and alternatives are required.

One key advantage of introducing diagnostic radiographer independent prescribers would be to enable them to write patient-specific directions to allow other, non-prescribing radiographers to administer the required medicines (such as contrast agents). Indeed, the absence of statutory exemptions for radiographers appears to add to the difficulty and makes clear the case for considering the use of all available mechanisms for accessing and administering medicines that would allow the timely delivery of services for patients and reduce the burden on radiologists. To date, most of the experiences of prescribing in radiography have been through supplementary prescribing by therapeutic radiographers. Diagnostic radiographers have largely been unable to avail themselves of the right to prescribe via a clinical management plan (CMP), because the latter assumes a diagnosis has been made (by the physician who is a signatory to the CMP), whereas the work of the diagnostic radiographer is often concerned with establishing a diagnosis. They may, however, also use prescribing of medicines in imaging to establish the effectiveness of treatment and the progress of disease. However, the model of supplementary prescribing is not broadly applicable to the practice of diagnostic radiography and has therefore largely excluded them from prescribing activity.

Yet, the lack of current exposure to prescribing activity by diagnostic radiographers does not appear to suggest there is no need for it. There are obvious instances where, for example, diagnostic radiographers administer agents via a Hickman's line or where sonographers prescribe for the treatment of deep vein thrombosis, although these remain rare in practice.

One factor, which may militate against the granting of independent prescribing to diagnostic radiographers, is the concern over simultaneous prescription and administration of a medicine. However, the capacity of a diagnostic radiographer to use independent prescribing to authorise other non-prescribing colleagues to administer medicines would both solve the problem and reduce the need for a radiologist's intervention.

**Therapeutic Radiography** Prescribing in therapeutic radiography is primarily undertaken by review radiographers, responsible for supporting patients through a course of radiotherapy. Such a treatment usually takes place over a 6–8-week period and involves monitoring and managing care related to the side effects of radiation exposure. However, the vagaries of treatment outcomes may create problems when trying to work within the constraints of a CMP. For example, therapeutic radiographers may wish to prescribe for pain control, in order to manage the effects of the radiation treatment itself, rather than the cancer for which they are receiving it. To do this effectively, a pre-agreed CMP has usually been necessary. However, it is not always clear in advance which patients are likely to progress through their radiotherapy treatment according to plan and which will require adjustments and changes to be made along the way. This raises a dilemma—should a clinical management plan be constructed for every single patient, just in case it is needed? In reality, because they are time-consuming and may cause delays to treatment, CMPs are not always drawn up. Even when they are set up in advance, they will list specific medicines, thus removing the flexibility needed to adapt and change to another medicine should the patient respond poorly to a particular medicine, for example, a pain killer.

It is likely that the prescribing pattern for most review radiographers making the transition from supplementary to independent prescribing would remain the same. Many work within a site-specific area (such as head and neck, breast or prostate) and are likely to continue to prescribe those medicines that they currently use via CMPs. The added advantage of independent prescribing, therefore, will be in the flexibility to alter treatment, for example, to step up the pain management ladder where and when necessary.


## 6.8    Undergraduate Education in Allied Health Prescribing: A Future Scenario?

At present, entry to AHP NMP programmes requires 3 years of postgraduate experience, and each programme has been designed with mainly specialist practitioners in mind, catering for those who are already working within a specific area of practice where prescribing is focused and where the applicants are deemed sufficiently advanced to be able to undertake prescribing safely and effectively.

However, it is not entirely inconceivable that in the future, prescribing by allied health practitioners might be established at undergraduate level, particularly given the fact that some professions, such as podiatry and optometry, currently access prescription-only medicines for supply and administration via statutory exemptions at that stage. Whilst there are no apparent plans to change the current system, it is worth considering the possible implications for future practice should such a shift occur. It might reasonably be argued that such a transition would essentially be evolutionary rather than revolutionary. If, for example, the programme were to be redesigned along the lines of a clinical clerking model, podiatrists and physiotherapists would be exposed to a deeper learning across the full range of body systems.

Such a system would have the potential to enable allied health practitioners to assume the role of DMP in the future and also to have more confidence in managing patients with multiple comorbidities. This would accord with the broader workforce redesign agenda and arguably relieve the heavy burden on hard-pressed physicians. It might also enable the allied health professions to contribute more obviously to creating and establishing a sustainable health service, building up a reserve of expertise which would be able to draw upon a broader appreciation and knowledge in managing patients pharmacologically, plus creating a resource over time of case histories and published research, and even leading to an involvement in the management of clinical trials of medicines.

## 6.9 Conclusion

A further formal scoping project has been launched to explore the need for prescribing, administration and supply mechanisms for the remaining allied health professions who as yet do not have prescribing rights. In addition, the Society and College of Radiographers (and, indeed, the College of Paramedics) is likely to explore opportunities for a resubmission to the Committee for Human Medicines for further consideration of the case for independent prescribing by diagnostic radiographers and also by paramedics. Intriguingly, most of the proposals for allied health prescribing first outlined in the Crown Report of 1999 have now come to fruition (Department of Health 1999). Its original intention was to broaden prescribing activity safely to those professions deemed able to contribute to the medicines management of their patients in a more effective way and to reduce the burden of prescribing on their medical colleagues. Although the formal evaluation being completed by the universities of Surrey and Brighton will provide the substantive evidence, the snapshot from practice offered in this chapter strongly suggests that AHP prescribing is making a difference, although not without complications and ongoing obstacles to the fulfilment of its full potential. It is at least clear that enabling the allied health professions to undertake the prescribing of medicines alongside their nurse and doctor colleagues affords their patients greater choice and speedier access to much needed medicines, in a healthcare system that is facing a growing demand for its services.

# References

AHPF (2013a) Outline curriculum framework for education programmes to prepare physiotherapists and podiatrists as independent/supplementary prescribers and to prepare radiographers as supplementary prescribers. A. H. P. Federation, London

AHPF (2013b) Outline curriculum framework for conversion programmes to prepare physiotherapist and podiatrist supplementary prescribers as independent prescribers. A. H. P. Federation, London

Borthwick A (2008) Professions allied to medicine and prescribing. In: Nolan P, Bradley E (eds) Non-medical prescribing—multi-disciplinary perspectives. Cambridge University Press, Cambridge, pp 133–164

Borthwick A (2012) A long and winding road: attaining independent prescribing rights for podiatrists. Diabetic Foot J 15(3):97–98

Borthwick A (2013) Independent prescribing: where are we now? Podiatry Now 16(4):2

Borthwick A, Short A, Nancarrow SA, Boyce RA (2010) Non-medical prescribing in Australasia and the UK: the case of podiatry. J Foot Ankle Res 3:1

Boyce R (2006) Emerging from the shadow of medicine: allied health as a 'profession community' subculture. Health Sociol Rev 15(5):520–533

Davies C (2003) The future health workforce. Palgrave MacMillan, Basingstoke

Department of Health (1999) Final report of the review of prescribing, supply and administration of medicines (Crown Report). Department of Health, London

Department of Health (2005) Supplementary prescribing by nurses, pharmacists, chiropodists/podiatrists, physiotherapists and radiographers within the NHS in England. Department of Health, London

Duckett S (2005) Health workforce redesign for the 21st century. Aust Health Rev 29(2):201

Freidson E (1988) Profession of medicine—a study of the sociology of applied knowledge. University of Chicago Press, London

Freidson E (2001) Professionalism: the third logic. Oxford University Press, Oxford

Hogg P, Hogg D (2006) Prescription, supply and administration of drugs in diagnosis and therapy. Synergy News (March Issue): 4–8

Hogg P et al (2007) Prescription, supply and administration of medicines in radiography: current position and future directions. Synergy News—Imaging and Therapy Practice (December): 26–31

Larkin G (1983) Occupational monopoly and modern medicine. Tavistock, London

Larkin G (1988) Medical dominance in Britain: image and historical reality. Millbank Q 66(Suppl 2):117–132

Larkin G (1993) Continuity in change: medical dominance in the United Kingdom. In: Hafferty W, JB MK (eds) The changing medical profession: an international perspective. Oxford University Press, Oxford

Larkin G (1995) State control and the health professions in the United Kingdom: historical perspectives. In: Johnson T, Larkin G, Saks M (eds) Health professions and the state in Europe. Routledge, London

Larkin G (2002) Regulating the professions allied to medicine. In: Allsop J, Saks M (eds) Regulating the health professions. Sage, London

Saks M (2013) The limitations of the Anglo-American sociology of the professions: a critique of the current neo-weberian orthodoxy. Knowl, Work Soc 1(1):13–31

Saks M (2014) Regulating the English healthcare professions: zoos, circuses or safari parks? J Prof Organ 1:84–98

# Part III
# The Practice, Art and Discipline(s) of Non-medical Prescribing

# Chapter 7
# The Identity of Non-medical Prescribers

**Sally Jarmain**

**Abstract** I still remember clearly how very exciting it was to become a non-medical prescriber. I was among the first tranche of nurses to train as independent prescribers, and it felt as though we were riding on the crest of a wave of innovation that would sweep through the health service. I finished the course with my head abuzz with new words—first-pass metabolism, partial agonists and bioavailability—ready to share my learning with patients and colleagues alike. At the time, I recall sitting down with a good friend of mine, discussing my new role over a few drinks in the pub. He was a medical consultant whose opinion I very much respected, and he told me in no uncertain terms that what I was doing was dangerous. How could I possibly diagnose conditions and prescribe for them without medical training? It is with some delight that I have read the literature pertaining to non-medical prescribing that has been produced since that time.

S. Jarmain
Northern Devon Healthcare Trust, Barnstaple, UK
e-mail: sally.jarmain@nhs.net

© Springer International Publishing AG 2017
P.M. Franklin (ed.), *Non-medical Prescribing in the United Kingdom*,
DOI 10.1007/978-3-319-53324-7_7

**Keywords**  Patient care • Clinical specialist independent non-medical prescribers • Electronic health records • Consultation • Therapeutic relationship • Shared decision-making • Concordance

## 7.1   Introduction

Not only has non-medical prescribing been demonstrated to be safe and clinically appropriate (Latter et al. 2012), but it is also cost-effective (i5 Health 2015), highly rated by patients (Courtenay et al. 2009) and accepted by other health professionals (Funnell et al. 2014). Even by my consultant friend, although that took a few years! Once I became a non-medical prescriber, my manager suggested that I move my desk into the office where the doctors were based. The reason given was that the computer, which was used to print out prescriptions, was in that room. Prior to taking on my new role, I had spent a vast amount of time waiting outside this office, so much so that I knew the pattern engrained in the wooden door intimately. I would stand and wait, whiling my time away, for the doctors to finish their important business. Eventually I would be admitted, with my request for a prescription.

Initially I felt that it was a good idea to move my desk, professedly for the same reason as my manager gave. Secretly, I felt that this move was an acknowledgement of my new, elevated position. What I did not understand at the time is that it moved me away from my existing professional support networks. Previously my desk had been in a large office full of nurses with whom I had identified closely. The doctors in my new office tried to be friendly and inclusive, but I was acutely aware of the fact that we were different. I was a non-medical prescriber, my very role by definition the antithesis of a medical prescriber. It was at this time that I experienced somewhat of a professional identity crisis. I felt strongly that I could provide better patient care as a result of my training. I was excited at what the future might hold for me professionally and the challenges ahead. However, I was scared of getting things wrong and I felt isolated in my new role. Imagine my surprise when a decade later a non-medical prescriber showed me the diagram in Fig. 7.1, as a pictorial representation of her identity. The feelings described in the diagram matched those of my earlier self precisely.

I am now employed as a non-medical prescribing lead, and a large part of my role is to support the non-medical prescribers in my organisation. I realised that I could not do this without fully understanding and appreciating how they viewed their identity. I wanted to find some way of doing this creatively. With this in mind, I decided to run a session on identity using a technique called the social photo-matrix (SPM) developed by

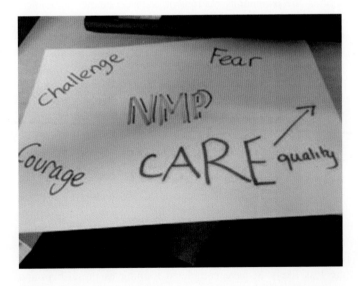

Fig. 7.1

Sievers (2008). This chapter will describe the technique and the subsequent results as a way of gaining deeper insight into the identity of non-medical prescribers.

## 7.2    Local Context

The organisation in which the SPM was conducted is a NHS Trust based in the South West of England. It covers around 2000 square miles, much of which is rural. The trust employs approximately 5000 staff. It includes an acute hospital with 450 beds, 17 community hospitals and a variety of community health- and social care services. There are 85 non-medical prescribers employed by the trust, 73 of whom are nurses. Half of the non-medical prescribers are community matrons or nurses, a quarter are clinical specialists and the remainder work within areas such as walk-in centres or accident and emergency departments.

There has been an interesting shift within the organisation, over the past 5 years; the number of community nurse prescribers has fallen, while the number of clinical specialist independent non-medical prescribers has grown. The former is of concern, given the current governmental emphasis on providing care closer to home (DH 2014). One reason for the reduction in community nurse prescribers is likely to be their age profile. A survey commissioned the Royal College of Nursing found that the average age of a community nurse was 46 years, with 35% of community nurse respondents aged 50 or older (Ball et al. 2014). Within my organisation, many community nurse prescribers completed the V100 prescribing course when they trained as district nurses in the 1990s. These nurses are now coming up to retirement age. The younger community nurses are less likely to have completed training as prescribers and sometimes question its benefit. Although the government has made a commitment to integrated electronic health records by

2020 (National Information Board 2014), this is not yet in place locally. As such, the community nurses often find it easier and safer to obtain the prescription items that they need through the GP surgery as opposed to prescribing themselves.

Alongside the reduction in community nurse prescribers locally, there has been an increase in the number of clinical specialists completing the non-medical prescribing course. Many of these cover both in-patient and community services, working closely with medical colleagues and providing advice/education within their area of expertise. In the first few years of its implementation, non-medical prescribing was taken up predominantly by individuals working in primary care or community settings (Courtenay et al. 2012). Within my organisation, it is therefore interesting to note its recent expansion into other specialties.

## 7.3   Social Photo-Matrix

There were varying responses from non-medical prescribers to my suggestion that we use the SPM tool. These included interest, amusement, disbelief and derision. This experiential methodology is potentially very challenging as it is designed to reveal the unconscious of an organisation. Most workplace practices are structured around the rational as opposed to the emotional (Vince and Broussine 1996), and any deviation from this can feel disconcerting. I had worries that nobody would attend the session and was enormously grateful to the 20 non-medical prescribers who withheld their judgement, parked their cynicism at the door and agreed to participate on the day!

So how does the SPM work? In the week preceding the session, I asked non-medical prescribers to take five photos that described their identity. They sent these to me and I randomly picked ten of the photos to display during the SPM. When they arrived at the session, the non-medical prescribers took their seats in a matrix formation (as defined by Lawrence 2005); each participant could view a large screen at the front of the room, but none of the participants could make eye contact with each other. The lights were dimmed and each of the ten photos was displayed for 5 min. While viewing the photos, non-medical prescribers called out words or phrases using the psychoanalytic methods of free association and amplification. Immediately following the SPM, there was a reflective session to discuss key emerging themes. These themes, and the photos that elicited them, will now be discussed.

## 7.4   Accountability and Governance

Many of the words and phrases that non-medical prescribers used when viewing the photo in Fig. 7.1 related to an awareness of the responsibility inherent within their extended roles. There was a sense of pride in their abilities, but also trepidation; *what happens if I get it wrong? Will I be supported?* In the reflective session that followed the SPM, non-medical prescribers talked of the need to abide by policies and procedures, both national and local. They were very aware of the governance structures in place within the organisation; in fact one of the other photos submitted was of the non-medical prescribing policy.

I was particularly interested in the anxiety that those present at the SPM experienced within their roles. As mentioned in the introduction to this chapter, fear was an emotion, which I too had experienced when I first qualified. However in my case this did not persist; once I had gained in confidence I no longer felt anxious. Many of the non-medical prescribers who attended the SPM had gained their qualification some time ago. It therefore intrigued and concerned me that in some cases a sense of anxiety remained for them, many years later.

Upon reflection I wonder whether the ongoing anxiety experienced by some non-medical prescribers is a symptom of the opposition that was so evident a decade ago. Unfortunately my consultant friend was not the only person to express concerns about non-medical prescribing. At the time of its introduction, the Chair of the British Medical Association vociferously opposed the change in legislation, expressing particular concern about the safety of allowing non-medics to diagnose conditions (Day 2005). This is relatively recent history. I might posit that non-medical prescribers still feel that they have something to prove to those who previously raised objections, and it is this that leads them to feel anxious.

## 7.5   Medicines Optimisation

A report by the Health and Social Care Information Centre (2015) found that the annual average number of prescriptions per head of population has increased from 13.7 items in 2004 to 19.1 items in 2014. Alongside this are the worrying findings that those diagnosed with multiple long-term conditions in the UK are increasing (the numbers are projected to rise from 1.9 million in 2008 to 2.9 million in 2018, DH 2012) and that 50% of those with long-term conditions do not take their medicines as prescribed (WHO 2003). The photo in Fig. 7.2 led non-medical prescribers in the SPM to talk about the issues that they faced, within this context.

Non-medical prescribers believed that they had a vital role to play in educating patients about their medicines, even if another prescriber had initiated these. They also talked about their function in stopping unnecessary prescriptions, which they viewed as being of equal importance to commencing prescriptions. Non-medical prescribers often have longer patient consultations than their medical colleagues, and they felt that the additional

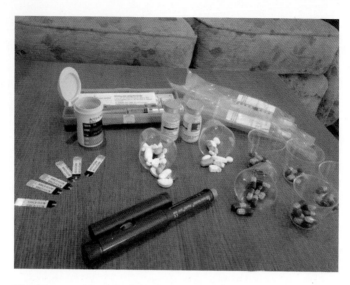

**Fig. 7.2**

time that they spent with their patients allowed them to discuss issues more thoroughly. It is interesting to note that while some studies have indicated that longer prescribing consultations lead to increased patient satisfaction (Seale et al. 2005), others have found that it is the content of the sessions (i.e. time spent describing treatment options) that is of greater significance in determining satisfaction (Weiss et al. 2014).

## 7.6   Therapeutic Relationship

In hospital, there are policies governing how medicines should be stored, temperature charts to record how cold the fridges are and infection control inspections to ensure that patients are not being put at risk. As the photo in Fig. 7.3 illustrates so accurately, this

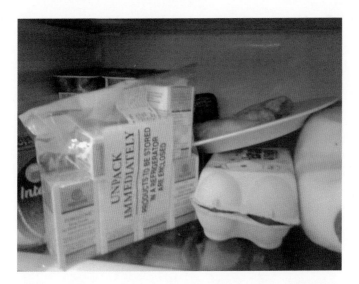

**Fig. 7.3**

is not necessarily the case within a patient's home! Non-medical prescribers who attended the SPM talked about how it is necessary for the patient and their prescriber to have non-judgmental conversations about how, when and where they take and store their medicines, in order to encourage honesty and, ultimately, concordance. They also talked about the need for creativity when considering options with patients, describing non-medical prescribing as being very much an art as opposed to a science.

Within the SPM and the reflective session that followed, non-medical prescribers talked about the therapeutic relationships that they build with their patients. They used words such as "holistic," "joint" and "shared." Weiss and Sutton (2009) argue that non-medical prescribers are further down the healthcare hierarchy than doctors. As such they may have a greater opportunity to develop a different kind of prescribing relationship, where true shared decision-making is perhaps more readily achievable.

## 7.7 Community/Hospital Prescribing

The idyllic scenery in Fig. 7.4 provides an example of the beauty inherent to the part of the country in which my organisation is based. The non-medical prescriber who took the photo told me that this is part of her *patch*, an area that she visits frequently for work. When I initially saw it, the photo prompted me to reflect on countryside walks and lazy summer days. However, the non-medical prescribers who attended the SPM were prompted to reflect on entirely different topics.

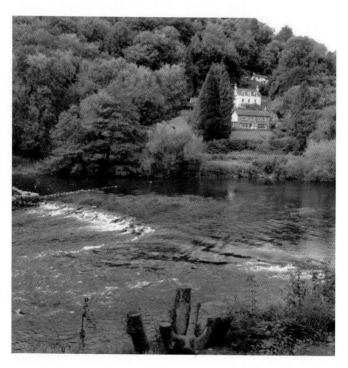

Fig. 7.4

They talked about the challenges of community work, attempting to reach an unwell patient in an isolated cottage through a raging snow storm, trying to negotiate an urgent supply of a medicine when the nearest pharmacy was many miles away and just about to close. Community non-medical prescribers are now handling these tasks, which would traditionally have fallen within the remit of the family doctor. The discussion on prescribing in the community led to an enhanced understanding of the differences between community and hospital work for those present. One of the hospital prescribers used an analogy that has remained with me ever since. She described non-medical prescribing as being like a tree; the roots are the same for all prescribers and consist of the content covered within the prescriber training such as pharmacology and consultation skills. However, the branches (i.e. the specialisms in which non-medical prescribers function) are multiple and diverse, and it is here that the power of non-medical prescribing lies.

Despite having different professional backgrounds and working in a variety of settings, I believe that there are some commonalities regarding the identity of non-medical prescribers that can be drawn from the SPM. Firstly, they all come from professional backgrounds that are further down the healthcare hierarchy than medical prescribers, and this may lead to different relationships with the patients for whom they prescribe. Secondly, they view their role in relation to medicines very holistically; it is not just about prescribing but also about educating patients on their medicines and stopping prescriptions where they are not needed. Finally, some non-medical prescribers continue to feel anxious about prescribing long after they have qualified. This fear of *getting things wrong* may hinder the implementation of non-medical prescribing within organisations and needs to be addressed through supportive organisational structures.

# References

Ball J, Philippou J, Pike G, Sethi G (2014) Survey of district and community nurses in 2013: report to the Royal College of nursing. NNRU, London

Courtenay M, Carey N, Stenner K (2009) Dermatology patients' views on nurse prescribers. Dermatol Nurs 8(2):38–44

Courtenay M, Carey N, Stenner K (2012) An overview of non-medical prescribing across one strategic health authority: a questionnaire survey. BMC Health Serv Res 12(138):1–13

Day M (2005) UK doctors protest at extension to nurses' prescribing powers. Br Med J 331:1159

Department of Health (2012) Long term conditions compendium of information, 3rd edn. The Stationery Office, London

Department of Health (2014) Five year forward view. The Stationery Office, London

Funnell F, Minns K, Reeves K (2014) Comparing nurses' and doctors' prescribing habits. Nurs Times 110(29):12–14

Health and Social Care Information Centre (2015) Prescriptions dispensed in the community 2004–2014. Available via http://content.digital.nhs.uk/catalogue/PUB17644/pres-disp-com-eng-2004-14-rep.pdf. Accessed 13 June 2017

i5 Health (2015) Non-medical prescribing—an economic evaluation. Health Education North West. Available via https://www.hee.nhs.uk/sites/default/files/documents/Agenda%20Item%207%20-%20i5%20Health%20-%20NMP%20Economic%20Evaluation.pdf. Accessed 22 Dec 2016

Latter S, Smith A, Blenkinsopp A et al (2012) Are nurse and pharmacist independent prescribers making clinically appropriate prescribing decisions? An analysis of consultations. J Health Serv Res Policy 17(3):149–156

Lawrence WG (2005) Introduction to social dreaming: transforming thinking. Karnac, London

National Information Board (2014) Personalised health and care 2020. Using data and technology to transform outcomes for patients and citizens: a framework for action. Available via https://www.gov.uk/government/publications/personalised-health-and-care-2020. Accessed 13 June 2017

Seale C, Anderson E, Kinnersley P (2005) Comparison of GP and nurse practitioner consultations: an observational study. Br J Gen Pract 55(521):938–943

Sievers B (2008) Perhaps it is the role of pictures to get in contact with the uncanny: the social photo-matrix as a method to promote understanding of the unconscious in organizations. Organ Soc Dyn 8(2):234–254

Vince R, Broussine M (1996) Paradox, defence and attachment: accessing and working with emotions and relations underlying organizational change. Org Stud 17(1):1–21

Weiss MC, Sutton J (2009) The changing nature of prescribing: pharmacists as prescribers and challenges to medical dominance. Sociol Health Illn 31(3):406–421

Weiss MC, Platt J, Riley R, Chewning B et al (2014) Medication decision making and patient outcomes in GP, nurse and pharmacist prescriber consultations. Prim Health Care Res Dev 16(5):513–527

World Health Organisation (2003) Adherence to long term therapies: evidence for action. World Health Organisation, Geneva

# Chapter 8
# Non-medical Prescribing
# in Community Settings

Sarah Kraszewski

**Abstract** Non-medical prescribing practice offers a wide
application to enhance practice in community and primary care
settings. This chapter briefly explores the origins and context of
non-medical prescribing amongst community professionals and
reviews examples of practice where the agendas have been successfully implemented. The evolving multi-professional teams
of prescribers in community practice influence the development
of timely, safe and effective care.

**Keywords** Community care • Primary care • Multi-
professional • General practice • Medicines optimisation • Medication Appropriateness Index (MAI) tool
• Outside the product licence • Mobile working • Specialist community public health nurses (SCPHNs) • Barriers to prescribing
• Electronic Prescribing Analysis and Cost (ePACT) data

S. Kraszewski
Anglia Ruskin University, Chelmsford, CM1 1SQ, United Kingdom
e-mail: sarah@krazz.co.uk

© Springer International Publishing AG 2017     145
P.M. Franklin (ed.), *Non-medical Prescribing in the United Kingdom*,
DOI 10.1007/978-3-319-53324-7_8

## 8.1  Introduction

The context of community prescribing care in the community is wide ranging, complex and delivered by a multi-professional team. Inevitably the supply and administration of medicines is a significant issue and one that can absorb a significant amount of time. There are a number of benefits relating to non-medical prescribers (NMPs) as part of the community team. It improves patient access to medicines, enables the medical team to spend more time focussing on complex cases and also supports professional autonomy amongst the NMPs, improving time management, as time is not wasted waiting for a general practitioner (GP) to sign a prescription (DH 2006). The activity and scope of NMPs in a community context is extensive. This ranges from both simple and complex nursing care in the home by community nursing teams to primary care provision offered in general practice and community healthcare settings. Furthermore, it includes services offered in the public health context, generated by encounters with health visitors (HVs) and school nurses or the amenities offered in community sexual health services.

Hart's (2013) study into the safety and effectiveness of independent prescribing activity amongst a group of community matrons demonstrates the diversity of their role and their contribution to the safe management of patients in a community setting. The matrons were undertaking a wide range of activity caring for older patients, including management of chronic obstructive pulmonary disease (COPD) exacerbation, cellulitis of the lower leg, urinary tract infections and pain management. She used the Medication Appropriateness Index (MAI) tool (also used by Latter et al. (2007) to appraise independent nurse prescriber activity) to evaluate medical prescriber's effectiveness. Whilst caution needs to be exercised in terms of sample size, Hart's findings were that the community matrons were prescribing appropriately and effectively and compared favourably with that published on the activity of general practitioners

(GPs). The success of the prescribing role of nurses has led the way for other professions and the implementation of new roles.

## 8.2  Medicines Optimisation

A key agenda for community prescribing practice is medicines optimisation and an area where NMPs working in community settings can have a huge impact. Medicines optimisation (MO) was introduced by the Royal Pharmaceutical Society in 2013 (RPS 2013) to help improve outcomes from medication use (Shah et al. 2014). There are many estimates as to how many medications are not taken as prescribed and that this can lead to adverse events and hospital admissions, as well as stockpiling in patient's cupboards. The community nursing workforce is working in the front line of caring for some of the most complex and vulnerable patients, for whom polypharmacy is a significant risk (Shah et al. 2014). NMPs can contribute greatly to improve the benefits, safety and value of medications to these patients.

The MO agenda encompasses four principles to support health professionals in facilitating patients to improve their quality of life and outcomes from medicines.

Principle 1:  Aim to understand the patient's experience.
Principle 2:  Evidence-based choice of medicines.
Principle 3:  Ensure medicine use is as safe as possible.
Principle 4:  Make medicines optimisation a part of routine practice.

The incorporation of these principles can be demonstrated via the following community scenario:

Prior to the rollout of independent prescribing, in order to dispense the necessary prescription-only medications (such as hormonal contraception or antibiotics to treat sexually transmitted infections), the community sexual and reproductive health (SRH) clinics relied upon either having doctors present at every clinic or the use of patient group directions (PGDs) by the nursing staff. The advent of independent prescribing rights for nurses has revolutionised the provision of such services, enabling the use of nurse-led clinics where the majority of clients' needs can be met efficiently by specialist nurses, utilising a hub and spoke approach for access to a doctor where clinically indicated. Clients (people attending sexual health service are usually referred to as 'clients' rather than the term 'patients' used in other services) presenting at these services often do so without prior records and with undifferentiated and undiagnosed needs. This requires skilled practitioners who can take a history, assess the client, formulate a diagnosis and prescribe treatment. In managing such scenarios, the practitioner needs to be able to understand the client's experience (principle 1) to enable the client to talk openly and achieve an agreed plan of treatment (e.g. the choice of contraception, ensuring it is something that is acceptable to the client and that they will be willing and able to use it). Any agreed plan of action (including a prescription) should be evidence based (principle 2) and cost-effective. In the case of a client enquiring about contraception, this will require the non-medical prescriber (NMP) to access the UK Medical Eligibility Criteria (UKMEC) for Contraceptive Use guidelines (FRSH 2016) as well as following guidance from local formularies and considering long-acting reversible contraception (LARC) (NICE 2014) methods. Safe use of medicines (principle 3) is incorporated into the history taking and use of appropriate decision-making tools and includes the counselling provided for the client. In this example, this may include the venous thrombosis risk associated with combined oral contraceptives (COC), potential interactions with other medicines now or in the future where other prescribers may be involved and the efficacy of the product selected.

The fourth principle, making MO part of routine care, is a core activity for any prescriber and in this scenario is about ensuring that the client can effectively use the chosen product, to obtain maximum efficacy and understand how it articulates with other current medications. The client should also remember to mention the use of the product in future consultations with other prescribers. The development of independent prescribing practice has benefited the care of clients in SRH services by providing the autonomy that the non-medical clinician requires. For example, if emergency contraception is required and the client does not fit neatly into the PGD (which may be for many reasons), a clinician who is not a prescriber cannot work outside the boundaries of a PGD. The NMP can, where they are happy to accept medicolegal responsibility and there is clear evidence supporting the use, prescribe 'off-label'. Prescribing off-label means that the prescriber is using a medication for an indication that sits outside the product licence or marketing authorisation. The independent prescriber may do so where it is in the best interests of the patient and that the available evidence supports such a decision. This type of activity is commonplace in some specialities such as paediatrics where there may not be appropriate formulations available (MHRA 2009). There are other examples, such as the use of a cycle or two of the combined oral contraceptive pill to regulate irregular bleeding experienced with contraceptive implants, which enables a NMP to provide complete patient care episodes within their scope of practice (NMC 2015).

## 8.3   Mobile Working

Mobile working describes the use of devices such as smartphones, laptops and other portable technology used to support clinical practice. As part of the *Transforming Community Services Programme* (DH 2011), a pilot study was undertaken to explore the benefits and challenges of mobile working and determine whether it was a worthwhile investment (Kidd 2011).

Four hundred clinicians from 11 NHS organisations participated and about 30% of these individuals were nurse prescribers. The project demonstrated that there were a number of benefits that emerged, particularly for nurse prescribers. Kidd (2011) reported these under several intersecting areas:

**Improved Access to Information**   For the nurse prescribers, remote access to clinical applications and the British National Formulary (BNF) and Nurse Prescribers Formulary (NPF) for Community Practitioners made a significant difference to their working day. It facilitated the completion of consultations and writing of prescriptions at the point of care.

**Increased Efficiency**   Administrative processes could be completed more efficiently. Where information sharing agreements were in place, it meant all information required to complete a care episode could be accessed (e.g. previous prescriptions, allergies, contraindications, results of tests). This also facilitated electronic prescribing (where the prescription is sent electronically to the pharmacy of the patient's choice) and made updating general practice records from the point of care a seamless process.

**Better Patient Contacts**   The nurse prescribers reported enhanced experiences when working with patients, as they were able to check information to provide reassurance (e.g. accessing discharge summaries to check a medication dose). The decision support applications (where the computer prompts the prescriber to check, e.g. allergies before prescribing) were seen by the nurses as a benefit and also support patient safety agendas.

**Improved Teamwork**   The mobile devices facilitated handover information and reduced travel times to and from base to collect information, as well as providing access to records from other clinicians involved in the patient care.

**Personal and Professional Benefits** The use of mobile working devices helped the clinicians to find new ways of working as well as increasing efficiency. It also aided the development of information technology skills, and the prescribing nurses felt this helped them to use their prescribing qualifications fully.

As with all mobile devices, some limitations such as poor quality signal necessitated individuals creating their own 'work-arounds', which whilst not ideal were necessary (e.g. such as saving data for entry until in a good reception area), but the participants still felt the benefits of the technology outweighed the limitations.

## 8.4   Community Formulary Prescribing by Specialist Community Public Health Nurses (SCPHNs)

Another public health area where prescribing by community practitioner nurse prescribers has a positive enhancement is that within the role of the health visitor and the school nurse. The majority of SCPHN courses include the v100 community practitioner's formulary prescribing qualification. This enables SCPHNs to prescribe from a limited formulary. Commonplace scenarios that SCPHNs may encounter where this can be beneficial include the management of oral candidiasis in infants (which if untreated may affect feeding and the wellbeing of the infant), bath and skin products to manage dry skin, management of head lice and smoking cessation products. By managing these and other common minor conditions, SCPHNs can ensure that individuals on their caseloads receive treatment in a timely fashion, can allay parental anxiety, save valuable GP appointments for more complex patients and achieve a satisfaction in their role brought about by the personal autonomy this can bring.

Furthermore, the delays in obtaining treatment where the SCPHN does not prescribe may not benefit patients, and some patients may not be able to afford over-the-counter treatments.

In many areas, it is known that there is a limited approach to health visitor prescribing. Thurtle (2007) undertook a study into establishing the reasons why health visitors (HVs) had lower prescribing rates than, for example, district nurses. Her study was undertaken in a London primary care trust and noted that the 'shared values, structure and strategy' were as important in establishing and sustaining a prescribing workforce as the expertise and attitudes of the prescribers. Whilst the majority of the practitioners surveyed were positive about prescribing, very few actually prescribed, citing difficult working contexts, the fact that many other issues take precedence and organisational systems that were not supportive of prescribing practice. There was no evidence of a culture of prescribing practice (Thurtle 2007). Unfortunately, whilst there has been some progress and champions who embrace prescribing practice, in the HV workforce active prescribers are in the minority, and this means that pressure continues on other services such as GP appointments for minor conditions that a health visitor (HV) might have treated. Thurtle's research made a number of recommendations, some of which are now evident in the modern community organisations, such as having an identified prescribing lead, streamlining of systems to obtain a prescribing pad on qualification and creating a non-medical prescribing strategy and programmes for continuing professional development (CPD). Many community formulary prescribers struggle to access appropriate CPD, and there is great variability in the local approaches to CPD for prescribers. It is difficult to ascertain whether prescribing features in the appraisal system for all HVs or just those who champion prescribing via their active use of the skill and qualification.

Hall et al. (2006) investigated why trained community nurse prescribers don't prescribe and identified a number of barriers:

Those that prevented prescribing (no prescription pad, no patient contact role, opposition from GPs and lack of confidence)

Those that prevented some prescribing (lack of time in clinics, access to prescribing budgets, security concerns, lack of access to patient records and alternative methods of supply)

Those that made prescribing more difficult, including record keeping, informing GP, delivering items to housebound patients and situations involving multiple prescribers

The above barriers, identified in 2006, are still in evidence today in some areas. It is interesting to note that in some respects, where community prescribing has been most successful, it is in the area of legitimising practice. For many years, GPs had signed prepared prescriptions for dressings for community nurses and other items such as contraceptive pills for practice nurses. As the nurses already felt confident in the use of such items, the impact of change on their confidence in their clinical decision-making when they qualify as prescribers is minimal (Hall et al. 2006). Hall et al. (2006) recommend that healthcare organisations need to monitor the prescribing activity to ensure appropriate support and encouragement is targeted where needed. Furthermore, they recommended developing approaches to integrate the non-medical prescribers into the wider healthcare teams to improve access to patients notes and the quality of the prescribing process (Hall et al. 2006). Monitoring of prescribing activity can be undertaken via Electronic Prescribing Analysis and Cost (ePACT) data, which is an electronic service holding *60 months of prescribing data on the NHS Prescription Services Database and is updated monthly* (NHSBSA 2016). It is worth noting that the decision not to prescribe can be as important as the one to prescribe, and alternative options such as over-the-counter purchase are also facilitated by competent prescribers.

Franklin (2006) raises the issues around whether the Community Nurse Prescribers' Formulary is fit for purpose given that the medications contained are mainly one-off treatments for minor conditions and can in the main be purchased over the counter. Certainly for district nursing teams, the wound care products are useful. The Community Nurse Prescribers' Formulary has remained a fairly static publication, without new additions, but is a useful adjunct to practice in particular areas such as wound care, minor conditions and smoking cessation.

## 8.5 Decision Making in Community Nursing

Luker et al. (1998) undertook an evaluation of community nurse prescribing. One of the key factors they identified was the decision-making process. They considered the models usually cited by the nursing literature such as the scientific approach versus the intuitive approach and discussed the potential influences such as the pharmaceutical industry, the patient, and the influence of nurses' own attitudes, that of colleagues' and that of their relatives'. Their findings confirmed that certain areas caused more anxiety, such as an element of uncertainty over a diagnosis, or a less familiar area of practice. Luker (1998) describes this in a simpler way: that district nurses seemed to be more comfortable about prescribing something they put on a patient (such as a dressing) rather then something they would put in a patient (such as a laxative). Many of the nurses expressed a need for more pharmacological training, something which has been addressed in the newer versions of the courses and as part of the NMC (2006) *Standards of Proficiency for Nurse and Midwife Prescribers*. Another identified aspect is the need for the community nurse prescribers to develop skills in managing uncertainty, which is something the independent prescribing students learn through their mentorship from medical colleagues. It could be argued that in many community situations, the full information is not available which can then impact on confidence to prescribe in less familiar situations. Community nurses are in a unique position as they tend to know their patients well and have contact with them more frequently than other professionals.

Dawson (2013) undertook an evaluation of the effectiveness of nurse prescribing in a community palliative care team. She undertook a small case study looking at how quickly patients received their medication after review by the clinical nurse specialist before and after the implementation of independent prescribing. The outcomes suggest that independent prescribing provided more timely access to medicines for this group of patients, which in turn means that patients may obtain effective symptom control and potentially be able to be able to receive end-of-life care in their preferred location, linking in with the updated NICE guidance on end-of-life care (NICE 2015).

## 8.6   Managing Long-Term Conditions in the Community

Non-medical prescribers working in community settings are well placed to support the management of long-term conditions (LTCs). Nurses have led the way in primary care in terms of developing extended roles through their activity in establishing nurse-led services for a range of LTC such as diabetes, asthma and COPD. Prescribing qualifications have enhanced this, enabling practitioners to complete their own consultations. Other professions are now following in the nurses' footsteps.

New initiatives to support the work of general practices include the recruitment of pharmacists to work in general practice, to alleviate the work of the general practitioner (NHS

England 2015). The pharmacists are now undertaking training in assessment and diagnostic skills and non-medical prescribing, to enable them to undertake management of long-term conditions such as asthma and COPD, field queries, optimise the use of medicines to reduce wastage, manage medications in terms of hospital discharges and repeat prescriptions and liaise between hospital pharmacies, community pharmacies, care homes and the general practice. The training is being facilitated by the Centre for Post Graduate Pharmacy Education (CPPE), and the pilots have commenced. Other pharmacist roles that are developing are those in the management of minor illness. In Essex, a recent pilot of a bespoke short course in minor illness management for community pharmacists was well evaluated by the participants (contact S. Kraszewski). Further evaluation is required to see if this then reduces attendance at general practice.

## 8.7    Conclusion

The evolution of multi-professional prescribing teams in the community setting continues to gather pace. Whilst it may not be necessary or desirable for every professional to train as a prescriber, the placement of key individuals has demonstrated a positive impact on the delivery of safe, effective and economical cost of care. This supports a skill-mix approach to ensure that the patient or client sees the most appropriate clinician, that the doctor's time is spent with the most complex cases and that care can be delivered closer to home. To continue this momentum requires the commitment of employers to support staff undertaking this training, both financially and in terms of flexibility to be able to take time for study and updating.

# References

Dawson S (2013) Evaluation of nurse prescribing in a community palliative care team. Nurse Prescribing 11(5):246–249

Department of Health (2006) Improving patients access to medicines. A guide to implementing nurse and pharmacist independent prescribing within the NHS in England. Available via http://webarchive.nationalarchives.gov.uk/20130107105354/http://www.dh.gov.uk/prod_consum_dh/groups/dh_digitalassets/@dh/@en/documents/digitalasset/dh_4133747.pdf. Accessed 22 Dec 2016

Department of Health (2011) Transforming community services. HMSO, London

Faculty of Reproductive and Sexual Health (2016) United Kingdom medical eligibility criteria for contraceptive use. Available via http://www.fsrh.org/site-search/?keywords=Faculty+of+Reproductive+and+Sexual+Health+%282016%29+United+Kingdom+medical+Eligibility+Criteria+for+Contraceptive+Use+. Accessed 22 Dec 2016

Franklin P (2006) Non-medical prescribing and the community practitioner: fit for purpose? Community Pract 79(12):388–391

Hall J, Cantrill J, Noyce P (2006) Why don't trained community nurse prescribers prescribe? J Clin Nurs 15:403–412

Hart M (2013) Investigating the progress of community matron prescribing. Prim Health Care 23(2):26–30

Kidd R (2011) Benefits of mobile working for community nurse prescribers. Nurs Stand 25(42):56–60

Latter S, Maben J, Myall M et al (2007) Evaluating the clinical appropriateness of nurses' prescribing practice: method development and findings from an expert panel analysis. Qual Saf Health Care 16(6):415–421

Luker K, Hogg C, Austin L et al (1998) Decision-making: the context of nurse prescribing. J Adv Nurs 2:657–665

Medicines and Healthcare Regulatory Agency (2009) Off-label or unlicensed use of medicines: prescribers' responsibilities 16. Available via https://www.gov.uk/drug-safety-update/off-label-or-unlicensed-use-of-medicines-prescribers-responsibilities. Accessed 14 June 2017

National Institute for Health and Clinical Excellence NG31 (2015) Care of dying adults in the last days of life. Available via https://www.nice.org.uk/guidance/ng31. Accessed 14 June 2017

National Institute for Health and Clinical Excellence (2005, updated 2014) Long acting reversible contraception CG30. Available via https://www.nice.org.uk/guidance/cg30. Accessed 22 Dec 2016

NHSBSA (2016) Electronic Prescribing Analysis and Cost (ePACT). Available via https://www.nhsbsa.nhs.uk/prescription-data/dispensing-data/information-services-prescription-cost-analysis-pca-data. Accessed 14 June 2017

NHS England (2015) News: new £15m scheme to give patients pharmacist support in GP surgeries. Available via https://www.england.nhs.uk/2015/07/pharm-supp-gp-surgeries/. Accessed 22 Dec 2016

Nursing and Midwifery Council (2015) The code: professional standards of practice and behaviour for nurses and midwives. Available via https://www.nmc.org.uk/standards/code/. Accessed 14 June 2017

NMC (2006) Standards of Proficiency for Nurse and Midwife Prescribers Available via www.nmc.org.uk/standards/additional-standards/standards-of-proficiency-for-nurse-andmidwife-prescribers/. Accessed 22 Dec 2016

Pharmaceutical Services Negotiating Committee (2016) Who can prescribe what? Available via http://psnc.org.uk/dispensing-supply/receiving-a-prescription/who-can-prescribe-what/. Accessed 22 Dec 2016

Royal Pharmaceutical Society (2013) Medicines optimisation: helping patients to make the most of medicines. Available via https://www.rpharms.com/promoting-pharmacy-pdfs/helping-patients-make-the-most-of-their-medicines.pdf. Accessed 22 Dec 2016

Shah C, Lehman H, Richardson S (2014) Medicines optimisation: an agenda for community nursing. J Community Nurs 28(3):82–85

Thurtle V (2007) Challenges in health visitor prescribing in a London primary care trust. Community Pract 80(11):26–30

# Chapter 9
# Prescribing for Long-Term Conditions

**Helen Skinner**

**Abstract** This chapter will discuss some of the issues surrounding prescribing within the field of long-term conditions. The chapter is divided into three sections:

(1) The relevance of compassion in practice relating to prescribing in long-term conditions and how the use of this can act as a safety net for the patient.
(2) The significance of the consultation and history taking. The approach the prescriber takes for both of these is key to forming a relationship with the patient and understanding personal health beliefs and goals.
(3) Issues around adherence, compliance, and concordance are explored polypharmacy and de-prescribing are also addressed.

**Keywords** Long-term condition • Communication Concordance • Adherence • De-prescribing

H. Skinner
Torbay and South Devon NHS Foundation Trust,
Bay House, Nicholson Rd, Torquay TQ2 7TD, UK
e-mail: helen.skinner3@nhs.net

© Springer International Publishing AG 2017
P.M. Franklin (ed.), *Non-medical Prescribing in the United Kingdom*,
DOI 10.1007/978-3-319-53324-7_9

## 9.1 Introduction

A long-term condition (LTC) is defined as a health problem, which cannot be cured and requires long-term treatment or therapy to control the symptoms (House of Commons 2014). LTCs have been of concern to healthcare providers for decades, and there are now an increasing number of people living with several LTCs—these people often have poor quality of life and longer hospital stays (Goodwin et al. 2010).

Modern management of patients with LTCs often requires input from clinicians skilled in the speciality. The doctor may not always be available at the point where a medicine needs introducing; thus, there may be a delay in treatment; access to other medical professionals qualified in prescribing widens the access to appropriate medications for the patient (Carey 2011). There is also strong evidence that people with LTCs feel that they are more involved in their consultations with nurse prescribers and thus better educated about their condition and supported to self-manage their own health (Courtenay et al. 2011; Stenner et al. 2011; Royal College of Nursing [RCN] 2012).

The relationship between the patient with an LTC and the prescriber—medical or non-medical—may be viewed as a journey, and making a difference for the patient is reliant on the ability to communicate with care and discernment (Balzer Riley 2016). Alongside of the inquiry into failings in Mid Staffordshire, chaired by Robert Francis (2013), the initiative of compassion in practice (Department of Health [DH] 2012) was implemented within the health service. A conscious effort on the part of the prescriber to uphold this approach may be key to effective treatment for the individual with an LTC. These principles should also strengthen individual professional prescribing development by informing the process of reflection.

Non-medical prescribers who work in a specialist field may only be responsible for managing one condition; however, consideration must be given to interactions with medication, which

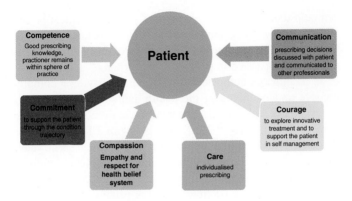

**Fig. 9.1**  Compassion in prescribing practice

are prescribed by other practitioners. It may be challenging to the prescriber to ensure that the medicines prescribed do not interact.

This chapter will explore some of the issues that arise in prescribing for people with long-term medical conditions (LTC). With our current ageing population, more people are living longer with one or more LTCs (LTC). This poses a challenge to the non-medical prescriber (NMP), as there may be complex interactions between the medications (Fig. 9.1).

Compassion in practice provides a model for non-medical prescribing in LTCs ensuring the patient remains central to the prescribing process.

## 9.2   Compassion in Prescribing Practice

Applying the principles of compassion in practice (DH 2012) to prescribing practice can be helpful in ensuring that the patient remains central to the process. Used alongside the competency framework (Royal Pharmaceutical Society (RPS) 2016), this can help the prescriber to ensure that personal practice is safe and effective while taking into consideration the individuality of the patient. This section of the chapter will take a brief look at applying compassion in practice to prescribing.

In healthcare, competence is defined as having a comprehensive understanding of the health and social requirements of the individual and the expertise to deliver care based on current evidence (DH 2012). People with LTCs should be diagnosed and treated by health professionals who have expertise in the speciality: furthermore, treatment should be in line with current national guidance (DH 2005). Prescribers who work in specialist fields are more likely to be working with drugs that are new to the market (Petty 2012); it is, therefore, important that these prescribers ensure they are kept up to date with information surrounding new medicines in their field; it is also important to participate in the reporting of adverse events.

Commitment to supporting the patient through the disease trajectory includes ensuring that the patient has access to timely support, advice is an important factor for people with long-term conditions and also helps adherence to treatment (Courtenay et al. 2011). Flexible appointments, telephone advice and continuity of care are all appreciated by patients and have been identified as contributing factors to improved outcomes (Carey 2011).

Respect and empathy for a patient's health belief system is fundamental to ensuring adherence to a course of treatment (Chummun and Bolan 2013). It is, therefore, imperative that the NMP explores the patient's viewpoint on any proposed treatment and supports the individual to make an informed choice giving the patient time to make a decision (Petty 2012). The prescriber should endeavour to build a trusting relationship with the patient (RPS 2016), and this should result in an open and honest consultation style with the patient feeling that they are fully involved in the decision-making.

Patients should be treated as an individual (Petty 2012). There are many issues that contribute to prescribing decisions including:

Age
Pregnancy
Cognitive ability/learning disability
Renal/hepatic function
Comorbidities

The prescriber should take these into consideration and ensure that the individual with an LTC is able to understand risk/benefit ratios and the aim of treatment (RPS 2016). There may be a requirement for in-depth counselling especially in the case of women of childbearing age. There may also be the need for mental capacity assessment and possible best interest decisions from the multidisciplinary team where the patient has been assessed as lacking capacity.

Supporting the patient with an LTC to self-manage their condition has long been advocated (DH 2005). Offering advice on lifestyle and other non-pharmaceutical methods of modifying disease is very much an integral part of the prescribing process (RPS 2016) and is particularly relevant to people with LTCs (Goodwin et al. 2010). Innovative treatments are also important in the management of LTCs, and although considered the province of specialists where this is within the competence of the prescriber, they should be offered to the patient (Petty 2012).

Well-developed communication skills are fundamental to the management of long-term conditions (Goodwin et al. 2010). For the prescriber, this means ensuring that the patient understands their treatment regime and where necessary providing written management plans to be followed. Communication with other members of the healthcare team is also important (RPS 2016)— especially with General Practitioners (GPs) who are often the first port of call for a worried patient. Where the patient has more than one co-existing LTC, communication between the multidisciplinary teams becomes even more significant to the patient well-being, and team meetings may be required frequently to ensure patient safety.

Using compassion in practice as a governance model in prescribing practice ensures that the patient remains central to the process, thus adhering to the values set out in the prescribing competency framework (RPS 2016). It can be used to form a safety net for both the patient with an LTC and the prescriber as it keeps the patient central to the prescribing process.

## 9.3   The Consultation

Improving the health and quality of life of the population should be at the centre of our prescribing practice. LTCs have become much more prevalent in our society as life expectancy has increased (House of Commons 2014). There are also several groups in society who require special consideration when prescribing, and these include the elderly, people with learning disability, women of childbearing age, and those with multiple long-term conditions.

The location of the initial consultation is often a practical decision; with early discharge from hospital targets, the initial consultation is more likely to take place in a clinic or the patient's own home. Other places such as day services, GP surgeries, or even the workplace may be appropriate dependent on the type of assessment necessary. Consideration may be given to whether bad news is given. Bad news is not limited to impending loss of life, but also may include the diagnosis in itself—for example, neurological conditions that are likely to inhibit lifestyle significantly and affect wider determinants of health such as mobility, social interaction, and employment (Parrott and Crook 2011; Silverman et al. 2013). Although little emphasis is given to the setting of the consultation, this is of significance for people with LTCs especially where this is associated with cognitive decline or physical and learning disabilities, and the following points may be useful to consider:

- Mobility
- Cognitive ability
- Physical constraints
- Environmental issues
- Witness accounts of symptoms
- Multi-professional involvement
- Breaking bad news
- Practitioner safety

Understanding the patient perspective and engaging the patient fully in decisions about treatment improve outcomes significantly (Last 2015). Thus, building a trusting compassionate relationship with the patient is likely to strongly influence the patient's perception of care (DH 2012). It is essential that the prescriber builds a relationship with the patient from the outset and this sometimes needs to include caregivers. A significant proportion of patients arrive at the consultation with their own ideas regarding the potential diagnosis and the implications of this. Listening to the patient's perspective should, therefore, be integral to the clinical assessment of the person with an LTC; this needs to be accepted and valued by the professional before a medical interpretation of the symptoms is offered (Silverman et al. 2013).

There is evidence that patients value discussing their condition with a health professional and emphasis of the risks and benefits of proposed treatments is considered especially important (Last 2015). When giving information about the treatment options, the prescriber also needs to include the option of no treatment and associated outcomes (RPS 2016). For some patients, this may be a real option dependent on the severity of their symptoms and the stage of the long-term condition, for example, early-stage Parkinson's disease. The trajectory and even the outcome of many long-term conditions may be modified by lifestyle or use of therapies (Box 9.1). The prescriber should be committed to understanding and discussing these topics with the patient and fostering a relationship where the prescription is not the only form of treatment considered (RPS 2016). Clinical experience reveals that discussions around possible treatment options can be protracted and may even need to be revisited over subsequent consultations. Commitment to gaining an understanding of the patient's health belief system and to achieving a plan of care and treatment based on a shared decision should therefore be the goal in management of LTCs.

---

**Box 9.1 Common Lifestyle Topics: This List of Lifestyle Topics Is Not Exhaustive and Prescribers Are Advised to Thoroughly Research Implications for Their Own Sphere of Practice**

**History Taking**
   Diet
   Alcohol
   Smoking
   Recreational drugs/substances
   Exercise/sporting activities
   Sleep deprivation
   Complementary therapies/medicines
   Use of dietary supplements
   Hydrotherapy
   Physiotherapy
   Occupational therapy
   Speech and language therapy

While this is covered in detail in other sections of the book in LTC management, the following brief indicators may be useful.

All prescribing decisions need to be based on a detailed clinical history and examination of the patient, taking into consideration all current health and social influences surrounding the patient (NMC 2006).

History of the presenting condition—this is central to the diagnosis and correct treatment. In LTCs, the patient's and sometimes also the witness's 'story' needs to be told partly to unburden the individual and certainly to capture the symptoms. The prescriber requires well-honed listening skills to support this storytelling. Effective (McCabe and Timmins 2013), active (Purtillo et al. 2014) and attentive (Silverman et al. 2013) have all been used to describe that intricate method of understanding that healthcare professionals aspire to. Sometimes it is useful simply to lay down the pen and give the patient your undivided attention—before reflecting back the salient points as you record them. There is a patient-led initiative for the story to only be told once (DH 2012); thus, it is imperative for people with long-term conditions that the prescriber is attentive to detail and that this is clearly documented and (with patient consent) shared with other healthcare professionals.

Medication history—a significant number of people with LTCs have comorbidities, and this is particularly evident in the elderly (Goodwin et al. 2010). Patients may have a significant number of concomitant medications and this raises the possibility for interactions. Complementary and alternative medicines are becoming more popular and accessible and may interact with conventional medicine, for example, St. John's wort interacts with many medications used across a wide spectrum of LTCs (Washer 2009). The prescriber, therefore, should give specific consideration to all treatments and therapies being used by the patient.

Past medical history, social history, family history and appropriate examination of the patient will also form part of the assessment.

People with LTCs should have a care plan that is shared across the multidisciplinary/multi-agency team with the consent of the patient (DH 2005). Medication management should form part of this care plan and include regular medication and medicines to be taken on a 'when necessary' basis or to be taken or administered in an emergency situation. Where medication is prescribed to be administered by a third party such as a relative or carer in the emergency situation, the prescriber should have individual, appropriate education alongside specific detailed instructions. This is particularly useful in the management of epilepsy where patients are known to experience prolonged seizures.

## 9.4   Compliance, Adherence, and Concordance

In the context of prescribing the terms, compliance, adherence and concordance are all used to describe an approach adopted by the patient in agreeing to follow a treatment plan. The patient may simply unquestioningly agree to take medicines as prescribed by the professional—described as compliance. Adherence suggests an element of informed choice for the patient before agreeing to take medicines as prescribed. Concordance has been cited as the 'gold standard' where the patient is fully involved in discussing the choices of treatment and medication available before a prescription is made (Kaufman 2014). Chummun and Bolan (2013) suggest that patients are more likely to take medicines as prescribed if they consider them to be necessary for their well-being.

There is evidence that about 20% of people do not take their medication as prescribed (Petty 2012); furthermore, as many as 50% believe that prescribed medicines do not have a positive impact on their medical condition (Chummun and Bolan 2013). Many people with LTCs will agree to take a medication as prescribed within the consultation, but once at home and their condition stabilises, they may alter their dose or even stop taking the medication altogether without consulting a healthcare professional (Petty 2012). Patients with LTCs who do not take their medication as prescribed risk a significant deterioration in their health, and there is the additional consideration that this may ultimately result in avoidable hospital admissions with a cost implication for health services (Felzmann 2012). It is therefore essential that the prescriber forms a relationship with the patient with an LTC and gains an understanding of the influences that surround how an individual approaches their own treatment and make a shared decision (RPS 2016).

There may be times when shared decision-making proves difficult especially where there is a concern regarding an individual's cognitive ability. It may be the LTC itself, which is associated with cognitive impairment such as Alzheimer's or Parkinson's disease, epilepsy (where there may be fluctuating levels of cognition) or a pre-existing learning disability. Giving guidance and information when prescribing should therefore be taken into consideration (RPS 2016). A mental capacity assessment and best interests decision around prescribing and administration of medicines may be required before the prescription is issued. It may also help if an arrangement is made with the chemist to provide blister pack medication.

Non-adherence to medication regimens may not always be intentional (Chummun and Bolan 2013), and reasons may include not being able to afford the prescription charge, simply forgetting to take the medicine and misunderstanding instructions. The prescriber has a responsibility to ensure that the patient is provided with adequate information as to how to take the medicine and this may need to be as a written care plan. Where there is a concern about memory impeding adherence, the patient may be advised to set an alarm—in clinical practice advice to use a mobile phone alarm may be helpful; there are also dosette boxes available that have a built in clock with alarm. The prescriber should make every attempt to ensure that the patient is aware of conditions where prescriptions are free and where prepaid prescription charges may help with costs—further information is available on NHS Choices website.

## 9.5 Polypharmacy and De-prescribing

Polypharmacy has been defined as taking more than four different medicines on a daily basis (Walker 2013). While in some cases it may be necessary for an individual to be taking four or more medicines where a patient has one or more long-term conditions, the probability of inappropriate polypharmacy increases (Duerden et al. 2013).

Underdosing has been identified as a contributing factor to inappropriate polypharmacy (Halczli and Woolley 2013). In the field of epilepsy, this sometimes occurs when a patient has commenced on a drug that is subsequently found to be ineffective; a second, third and, rarely, even a fourth medication may be introduced in an attempt to control the symptoms without reducing and stopping any of the previous drugs. The difficulty is that this is not an exact science! Some patients may require polytherapy to control the seizures, while others may have ended up on combinations of drugs because their appointments are delayed or missed; or even because there is a change of prescriber during a change of drug. A contributing factor to the last is that many antiepileptic drugs need slow titration to ensure that the lowest effective dose is prescribed and also to increase tolerability.

Where the individual has more than one long-term condition, lack of co-ordination may contribute to inappropriate polypharmacy (Walker 2013). This is especially seen where an individual is receiving prescriptions from several health professionals. Adverse drug reactions (ADRs), interactions between medications and errors in taking medication as prescribed are all risks associated with polypharmacy (Walker 2013; Duerden et al. 2013). Prescribing as part of a team is always considered an aspect of good governance (RPS 2016); but where polypharmacy is considered necessary for the well-being of the patient, this takes on further significance. Suggestions for good team working are listed in Box 9.2.

> **Box 9.2 Managing Polypharmacy Through Team Working**
>
> Multidisciplinary team meetings and joint patient appointments.
> Co-ordination of care from one professional—usually GP.
> Pharmacist involvement.
> Inter-professional support and supervision.
> Ensure therapeutic dose is prescribed.
> Regular review.
> Support for caregivers.
> Use of dosette boxes or blister packs.

De-prescribing is a term that came into use in the first years of the twenty-first century to describe the process of reducing and/or stopping medicines that are no longer required (Frank 2014). The overarching aim of de-prescribing is to reduce polypharmacy harm and improve adherence to those medications necessary for the individual's well-being (Frank 2014). Anderson et al. (2014) found that prescribers find it difficult to reduce medications, and furthermore when a medicine is reduced and stopped, it is often recommended within a few months.

Patients themselves are frequently willing to consider de-prescribing but may lose confidence during the reduction or disagree about which medicine is the correct one to stop. Ensuring that the patient is well informed and supported throughout the de-prescribing process may in some measure mitigate these concerns (Reeve et al. 2014). Ensuring that the patient is directed to reliable sources of information about their medical condition(s) and ensuring that this is presented in a way that is understandable to the individual are integral parts of the prescribing process (RPS 2016). Reeve et al. (2014) have developed a patient-centred, five-step process for de-prescribing which is reflected by the six-step consultation process outlined in the prescribing framework (RPS 2016).

Because of complex interactions and adverse effects often associated with anti-epileptic medications, de-prescribing has become a routine element of my prescribing practice as an epilepsy specialist nurse. I have found that the key to success is the fifth stage—monitoring, support and review. Giving the patient an individual schedule to follow is valued by patients and helps to minimise errors. Also as it is frequently difficult to offer clinic appointment on a frequent basis, I support patients through telephone consultations during planned medication reductions. I find that negotiating frequency of these with the patient—usually beginning with weekly appointments and then reducing, as their confidence increases—is usually enough support through a potentially anxious time (Box 9.3).

> **Box 9.3 De-prescribing Process** (Reeve et al. 2014; RPS 2016)
>
> Assess the patient and take a full history with emphasis on medication.
>
> Discuss treatment option with the patient and identify medications that may be inappropriate.
>
> Reach a shared decision with the patient as to which medication can be reduced.
>
> Plan reduction and prescribe, providing the patient with a written schedule to follow.
>
> Monitor and review the patient.

## 9.6   Conclusion

This chapter has offered some general insights into prescribing in the field of LTCs. It is impossible to give specific advice for individual conditions in such a short chapter; thus, I have focussed on some general principles that can be applied to diverse conditions. I have found in my own practice that using the first consultation to take a comprehensive history is invaluable. Although it may require a longer appointment than usual, it often saves time and prevents misunderstanding later in the patient journey and can preserve the relationship between the professional and patient.

In my experience as an epilepsy nurse specialist, I have found that taking time to form a trusting relationship from the outset often helps to understand the situation from the individual patient perspective. This may well improve adherence and prepare the way for difficult conversations regarding de-prescribing where polypharmacy proves to be an issue.

Using the six Cs (DH 2012) as a governance framework in prescribing for long-term conditions supports the professional in keeping the patient central to the process. Competence, commitment, compassion, care, courage and communication can be used to encompass all the issues in prescribing and have natural links with the prescribing process when viewed alongside the prescribing competency framework (RPS 2016).

Finally, prescribers are all bound by the same principles; including their own professional body and employer's governance, and national and local guidance regardless of their field of practice; and the information contained in other chapters of this book may also be applied to LTCs. This chapter is not intended to cover all the issues that confront those prescribing for LTCs—but more to examine some of the more challenging aspects of this role.

# References

Anderson K, Stowasser D, Freeman, C et al (2014) Prescriber barriers and enablers to minimising potentially inappropriate medications in adults: a systematic review and thematic analysis. BMJ Open. Available via http://bmjopen.bmj.com/content/4/12/e006544.full. Accessed 23 Dec 2016

Balzer Riley J (2016) Communication in nursing, 8th edn. Elsevier, St Louis

Carey N (2011) Does non-medical prescribing make a difference to patients? Nurs Times 107(26):14–16

Chummun H, Bolan D (2013) How patient beliefs affect adherence to prescribed medication regimens. Br J Nurs 22(5):270–276

Courtenay M et al (2011) Patients views on nurse prescribing, effects on care, concordance and medicine taking. Br J Dermatol 164(2):396–401

Department of Health (2005) National service framework for long term conditions. The Stationery Office, London

Department of Health (2012) Compassion in practice. Nursing, midwifery and care staff our vision and strategy. Available via https://www.england.nhs.uk/wp-content/uploads/2012/12/compassion-in-practice.pdf. Accessed 23 Dec 2016

Duerden M, Avery T, Payne R (2013) Polypharmacy and medicines optimisation making it safe and sound. The Kings Fund, London

Felzmann H (2012) Adherence, compliance, and concordance: an ethical perspective. Nurse Prescribing 10(8):406–411

Francis R (2013) Report of the mid Staffordshire NHS trust public inquiry. Available via http://webarchive.nationalarchives.gov.uk/20150407084003/ and http://www.midstaffspublicinquiry.com/sites/default/files/report/Volume%201.pdf. Accessed 14 June 2017

Frank C (2014) De-prescribing: a new word to guide mediation review. Can Med Assoc J 186(6):407–408

Goodwin N et al (2010) Managing people with long term conditions. The Kings Fund, London

Halczli A, Woolley A (2013) Medication underdosing and underprescribing: issues that may contribute to polypharmacy, poor outcomes

House of Commons Health Committee (2014) Managing the care of people with long term health conditions. Second Report of Session 2014–15. Available via https://www.publications.parliament.uk/pa/cm201415/cmselect/cmhealth/401/40102.htm. Accessed 14 June 2017

Kaufman G (2014) Polypharmacy, medicines optimization and concordance. Nurse Prescribing 12(4):197–201

Last R (2015) Communicating with patients with long-term conditions. Pract Nurs 26(3):147–150

McCabe C, Timmins F (2013) Communication skills for nursing practice, 2nd edn. Palgrave, London

Nursing and Midwifery Council (2006) Standards of proficiency for nurse and midwife prescribers. Available via https://www.nmc.org.uk/standards/additional-standards/standards-of-proficiency-for-nurse-and-midwife-prescribers/. Accessed 14 June 2017

Parrott T, Crook G (2011) Effective communication skills for doctors. BPP Learning Media, London

Petty D (2012) Ten tips for safer prescribing by non-medical prescribers. Nurse Prescribing 10(5):251–256

Purtilo R et al (2014) Health professional and patient interaction, 8th edn. Elsevier, St Louis

Reeve E, Shakib S, Hendrix I et al (2014) Review of de-prescribing processes and development of an evidence-based, patient-centred de-prescribing process. Br J Pharmacol 78(4):738–747

Royal College of Nursing (2012) Factsheet: nurse prescribing in the UK. Available via https://www.rcn.org.uk/about-us/policy-briefings/pol-1512. Accessed 14 June 2017

Royal Pharmaceutical Society (2016) A competency framework for all prescribers. Available via https://www.rpharms.com/Portals/0/RPS%20document%20library/Open%20access/Professional%20standards/Prescribing%20competency%20framework/prescribing-competency-framework.pdf. Accessed 14 June 2017

Silverman J, Kurtz S, Draper J (2013) Skills for communicating with patients. Radcliffe Publishing, London

Stenner K et al (2011) Consultations between nurse prescribers and patients with diabetes in primary care. A qualitative study of patient views. Int J Nurs Stud 48(1):37–46

Walker T (2013) Lack of coordination, copious prescribing drive polypharmacy challenges. Formulary 48(2):83

Washer P (2009) Clinical communication skills. Oxford University Press, Oxford

# Chapter 10
# Non-medical Prescribing
# in the Acute Setting

**Jayne R. Worth**

**Abstract** Non-medical prescribing in the acute setting presents both challenge and opportunity. The challenge inherent within the remit of an advanced nurse practitioner in a Hospital at Night Team is to provide safe and effective care to deteriorating patients across a wide range of clinical specialties. The opportunity, is to apply the holism of nursing to a traditionally medical role. By facilitating the provision of seamless care from one healthcare professional, non-medical prescribing not only benefits patients by expediting treatment, by supporting the autonomy of advanced nursing practice it enhances job satisfaction. Whilst robust governance at national and local level is required to provide a benchmark for safe and effective practice, individual non-medical prescribers and their parent organisations hold a joint responsibility towards continuous professional development. Containing examples taken from the author's clinical practice and a small audit of her personal non-medical prescribing practice, this chapter aims to illustrate the role of non-medical prescribing in the acute setting. All identifiable patient details have been removed.

J.R. Worth
NHS Lothian, Edinburgh, UK
e-mail: jayne.worth@luht.scot.nhs.uk

© Springer International Publishing AG 2017      177
P.M. Franklin (ed.), *Non-medical Prescribing in the United Kingdom*,
DOI 10.1007/978-3-319-53324-7_10

**Keywords** Hospital at Night • Advanced nurse practitioner • Patient group direction (PGD) • Accountability • Liability • Remote prescribing • Shared care • Communication • Audit • Patient safety

## 10.1 Introduction

### 10.1.1 The Development of Non-medical Prescribing Within a Hospital at Night Team

The Hospital at Night Team (HAN) in Lothian covers three teaching hospitals ($n = 2020$ beds) offering a wide range of general and specialist services. Providing a service tailored to the needs of each hospital site, the team is comprised of senior and advanced nurse practitioners, foundation year one and two doctors, clinical development fellows and medical registrars with access to consultants on call.

The position of advanced nurse practitioner (ANP) within HAN can be demanding yet, both personally and professionally, very rewarding. The advanced practice role involves complex decision-making based upon structured patient history taking and clinical examination, the generation of differential diagnoses and the formation of management plans.

The majority of patients reviewed by ANPs are frail and elderly, with multiple comorbidities and little physiological reserve. Their clinical presentations are often atypical in nature and can be complicated by varying degrees of cognitive impairment and delirium. Conditions requiring prompt intervention, such as sepsis (severe infection), acute pulmonary oedema (fluid overload of the lungs) or atrial fibrillation (irregular heart rate), are encountered by ANPs on a nightly basis.

Whilst able to write up limited medications under a patient group direction (PGD), for example, simple analgesics, intravenous fluids and anti-emetics, the ANPs were unable to prescribe outwith the PGD formulary. As a result of this restriction, patients requiring escalation of analgesia, alteration of antibiotic doses following blood results or the prescription of routine medications that had been missed during the day, such as evening insulin doses or warfarin, did not always receive their medication at acceptable times of night.

In deteriorating situations, the restrictive nature of PGDs occasionally led to delays in the initiation of treatment as the patient had to wait for a medical review and subsequent prescription. This situation was highly frustrating for ANPs who had the knowledge and experience to treat acutely unwell patients, yet were unable to prescribe the appropriate medication. Achieving a qualification in non-medical prescribing (NMP) was the logical next step in the evolution of the advanced practice role.

NHS Lothian requires ANPs to successfully complete two master's level modules on patient history taking and clinical examination before embarking upon the NMP module. This is not true of all healthcare authorities, but, as this chapter aims to illustrate, in order to prescribe the correct drug, you must first reach the correct diagnosis.

As formal education at master's level involves a considerable investment of time and personal study over and above the clinical hours worked, it has a significant impact on work-life balance. A high level of commitment is required from ANPs to develop and subsequently maintain their skills as non-medical prescribers.

## 10.2 Accountability, Liability and Prescribing Formularies

According to the Nursing and Midwifery (NMC) Standard Number 2 for Non-medical Prescribing (2006), a non-medical prescriber must accept personal accountability for all aspects of her prescribing practice. NHS Lothian states it will hold vicarious liability at an organisational level as long as a non-medical prescriber prescribes within the parameters of the organisation's formulary.

An ANP's personal core formulary is a profile of the medications she has studied and feels competent in her knowledge and understanding, not only of the biochemical and physiological properties of the drugs: its pharmacokinetics (how the drug travels and is processed by the body) and its pharmacodynamics (the effects of the drug upon the body), but also in her judgement that the prescription is appropriate to the clinical situation.

ANPs in HAN are responsible for the care of patients across a wide range of general and specialist areas; the medications they are required to prescribe are also diverse. The generic nature of the role is a stark contrast to the NMP remit of ANPs working in specialist areas whose NMP practice is based around clearly defined protocols and small core formularies.

As will be discussed in Sect. 10.7, the individual nature of each ANP's core formulary has implications for continuing professional development (CPD). On occasion it has also resulted in a degree of misunderstanding from other healthcare professionals. Each ANP prescribes from within her own scope of competence which is strongly influenced by her clinical background, for example: coronary or intensive care, acute medicine or surgery. Therefore, there will be situations where an ANP will feel confident in her assessment and management to work autonomously yet in another may require assistance.

One example from practice is the treatment of a patient who has developed fast atrial fibrillation (AF) secondary to hypotension (low blood pressure) due to severe sepsis. In this context, the first response would be to prescribe intravenous fluids to restore haemodynamic (circulatory) stability. Continued fast AF despite fluid resuscitation would require treatment with antiarrhythmic medication to restore normal cardiac rhythm (Arrigo et al. 2014).

The prescribing decision required relates to which of the various classifications of antiarrhythmic medication is appropriate to the individual clinical situation. Whilst this decision would not be made in isolation, the prescription would be written by an ANP whose knowledge of cardiac drugs and their action made her confident to do so.

## 10.3   When Not to Prescribe

This aspect of the NMP role relates to circumstances where an ANP makes a decision not to prescribe a medication that has been requested. As previously stated, this not only depends upon an awareness of personal boundaries of knowledge and experience, it requires an understanding of the wider public health issues associated with the prescription request.

Antimicrobial stewardship is at the forefront of current healthcare policy (Colligan et al. 2015) and requires a prescribing decision based upon the best interests of the patient and the wider population. The interpretation of "best interests" often differs between healthcare professionals and patients. A request for a prescription of antimicrobials in a pyrexial but otherwise well patient is a common example of an inappropriate request and often requires the management of patient expectations due to misconceptions about the role and effectiveness of this class of drugs.

One further example of a common prescription decision faced by an ANP in HAN is a request for sedation for an agitated elderly patient. Due to the risk of potential harm from multiple side effects, best practice states it is safer to manage this group of patients using non-pharmacological measures (National Institute for Health and Care Excellence 2010). These measures include an assessment for precipitating factors such as pain, urinary retention or developing delirium plus management of the patient's environment. Sedation should only be prescribed when these measures have failed. Patients, relatives and nursing staff often need support and guidance to steer them through what can be a demanding situation for all concerned.

## 10.4   Remote Prescribing

The final prescribing aspect of the HAN non-medical prescriber is the generation of remote prescriptions. A remote prescription is one that is issued via email, telephone or by fax. This service is required of HAN as it provides remote cover to a small general hospital without medical cover overnight. As with all areas of nursing practice, there are guidelines to follow and standards to be met before a remote prescription can be generated (NMC 2008).

Once the senior nurse on the remote site has assessed the patient, she presents her clinical findings over the telephone, including details of the patient's anticipatory care plan and escalation status. This information is supplemented by accessing the patient's electronic records. Once sufficient information has been obtained, a non-medical prescriber, who judged it was within her scope of competence, would write the required prescription which would be sent electronically via email or directly to the patient's electronic records.

## 10.5   NMP in the Acute Setting

### 10.5.1   Case Study One

An 87-year-old male patient was referred to HAN as he was vomiting despite the administration of two different anti-emetics. Nursing staff were concerned the patient may have aspirated (inhaled) his vomit.

The patient was receiving intravenous fluids and antimicrobials for the treatment of aspiration pneumonia and laxatives for constipation. His medical history included a residual right hemiparesis (paralysis) and aphasia (inability to speak) following a stroke 8 years before and chronic obstructive airways disease (lung disease secondary to smoking).

A review of his vital signs showed he had a high temperature and rising heart rate. His blood pressure was stable at the time, but the levels of oxygen in his blood were starting to drift down, and his respiratory rate was trending up. A rising respiratory rate is one of the first indicators of clinical deterioration and may occur hours before an observable decline in a patient's condition is seen.

On examination the patient was found to be peripherally cold with mottling of his skin; he had increasing crepitations (crackles) in his right lung and new crepitations in his left lung. He continued to vomit dark, bilious liquid. He had no abdominal distension or obvious tenderness on palpation, and his bowel sounds were scant. His urine output had decreased markedly over the previous 10 hours.

The investigations ordered as part of the assessment of his physical condition indicated increasing levels of infection and inflammation. The appearance of increased consolidation (infection) on his chest X-ray indicated worsening pneumonia. Faecal loading with dilated gassy loops of the large bowel on his abdominal X-ray (AXR) suggested the possibility of the development of a bowel obstruction.

From the clinical examination and test results, a diagnosis of severe sepsis secondary to worsening pneumonia was made. The differential diagnosis was of an obstructed bowel as a result of either sepsis-induced multi-organ failure leading to paralysis of the smooth muscles of his small intestine or obstruction of his large intestine secondary to constipation.

A review of the patient's medical notes showed a documented plan for the addition of a further antibiotic to his current regime. This prescription required the use of a calculator, which computes the dose and dose interval for the drug using values including the patient's age, weight and creatinine clearance.

As the patient's blood pressure started to fall, an intravenous fluid bolus was prescribed with the aim of improving his circulating volume and supporting his renal function. The rate of his maintenance fluids was subsequently increased to replace the fluid losses that had occurred due to vomiting and fluid shifts within the body. Fluid is lost from the circulation to the tissues secondary to the physiological changes that occur within blood vessels as a result of sepsis and can lead to a relative hypovolaemia.

The patient was informed of the plan for his care, but his level of agreement was difficult to assess due to his aphasia and the severity of his illness.

## 10.5.2 Case Study Two

HAN was asked to chase blood results for a patient who had fallen earlier in the evening. He was 77 years old and had been admitted with a history of falls on a background of advanced hepatocellular malignancy (liver cancer) and haemachromatosis (high iron deposition leading to organ damage). His blood results showed a mild acute kidney injury with hyperkalaemia (elevated serum potassium level). Clinically, he was dehydrated with a poor oral intake.

A review of his medication Kardex showed no drugs that could potentially precipitate either a kidney injury or a high potassium level. Hyperkalaemia can lead to cardiac arrhythmias (abnormal heart rhythms) so an electrocardiogram was recorded (ECG). His ECG showed none of the changes that can occur in this instance. This is an important determinant of treatment, as, should there have been hyperkalaemic changes, the patient's treatment would have included the prescription of medication to stabilise his cardiac muscle, whilst his serum potassium was being returned to safe levels. The NMP decision was to treat with an insulin and dextrose infusion, as per treatment guidelines (British National Formulary 2016) along with intravenous fluids to support the patient's low oral intake.

This treatment plan was discussed with the patient, not only from the perspective of good practice, but following the provision of information by the patient's nurse stating that the patient had expresssed a wish to die. Further discussion with the patient elicited the information that he was scared to go home in case he fell again. He was a widower who lived alone and he wanted to die so he could be with his wife again. His mood was very low, and this was contributing towards his reduced oral intake, as, despite experiencing feelings of hunger and thirst, he felt no motivation to eat or drink.

After discussing the rationale behind the treatment of his hyperkalaemia and what the treatment involved, the insulin and dextrose infusion was administered. Intravenous fluids were commenced to support his oral intake in the short term, and a plan was made to recheck his bloods later in the night.

The intervention and discussion with the patient were clearly documented in the patient's medical notes and verbally handed over to the day team. This handover included issues to be taken forward during the day with respect to the management of his electrolytes, fluid balance, emotional state and plans for discharge.

## 10.6 Shared Care, Communication and the Importance of Good Documentation

A patient's engagement and compliance with treatment starts with their understanding of the associated risks and benefits of that treatment. A paradigm shift from prescriptive to collaborative care placed shared care at the heart of strategic policy-making at both national and organisational level (Scottish Government 2007).

With shared care, patients and healthcare staff share a common goal where patients are empowered to take responsibility for their health and treatment decisions. A patient's expectations and previous access to healthcare has an impact on their engagement with the concept of shared care. An effective non-medical prescriber has to ascertain and manage a patient's expectations for their treatment and be able to communicate those findings to the patient's healthcare team.

However, in acute situations such as case study one, where the patient was too unwell to make informed decisions about his care, issues such as capacity and consent are highly relevant, and legal safeguards are necessary to support and protect both staff and patients. Case study two illustrates how the traditional holism of nursing, with its associated skill of building a rapport with a patient over a short space of time, dovetails neatly with the concept of shared care.

Clear and concise communication is one factor without which the potential for error, misunderstanding and delays in treatment rises exponentially. From previous experience, suboptimal communication forms the basis of many of complaints about care. Regulatory bodies such as the NMC (2015) and local clinical governance policies set standards to support both staff and patients.

Both case studies illustrate the role of good documentation in supporting the provision of seamless care. In case study one, the documented escalation plan and discussion around ceiling of care expedited the decision-making required to plan his treatment. In case study two, concern about the extent of the patient's low mood was documented to inform the patient's own team and guide discussion and decision-making on future care needs.

Whilst patients who have been reviewed overnight are handed over to their respective day teams in the morning, it is often to one junior doctor from each clinical specialty who then feeds back to the other doctors in their area. This verbal chain of communication benefits greatly from a contemporaneous record of a NMP's assessment, decision-making process and the patient's response to the medication prescribed. Thus it can be said that there are both professional and practical reasons for good documentation.

## 10.7 Safe Practice

Autonomy and accountability walk hand in hand with the duty of care owed to patients to receive care based on evidence-based guidelines for best practice and to a standard required of professional bodies. However, autonomy does not equate with isolation and one of the key benefits of practising within the HAN team model is its teamworking philosophy. Whilst the ability to function within the team as an autonomous prescriber facilitates prompt response times, access to senior medical advice supports the delivery of safe and effective patient care.

Access to expertise also provides opportunities for learning, for reflective discussions on the management of deteriorating patients and supports CPD. Before a prescription is written, a non-medical prescriber must not only be competent to make the correct diagnosis; she must also have a sound working knowledge of the drugs that she wishes to prescribe (NMC Standard 3.3 2006).

It is neither possible nor advisable, to rely on memory when prescribing drugs. To support safe prescribing practice, factors such as age, renal and liver function, drug interactions and developments in best practice need to be taken into consideration. Recourse should be made to decision support tools such as the British National Formulary and reference made to local national guidelines and policies (National Prescribing Centre 2016). These resources not only provide information on best practice; they also disseminate alerts on emerging safety or recall issues. Access to the Internet and to email is required to receive those alerts, another resource consideration.

The safety of NMP has been demonstrated by reports such as the Scottish Government's (2009) evaluation of the safety profile of NMP in Scotland. This report provided reassuring evidence, not only that NMP was safe, it had a positive impact on patient satisfaction and access to treatment. NMP was beneficial in terms of professional satisfaction for non-medical prescribers and there was a definable public health impact in relation to antimicrobial stewardship. The barriers identified by the report were those which can be found in any large organisation—those of institutional and personal attitudes and the perennial issue of scarce resources.

## 10.8   Audit and CPD

It is a requirement of both governmental and nursing regulatory bodies for NMPs to continually evaluate their professional practice using reliable methods and to act upon their findings in order to improve their practice (NMC 2006). Robust guidelines and policies, access to continuing professional development (CPD) resources and an ongoing audit of prescribing practice are keystones of safe and effective NMP practice. Both individual NMP and health boards have a joint responsibility towards maintaining professional competence.

As part of their CPD, the ANPs run a continuous audit of their prescribing practice. The results of their personal audits can be discussed at their yearly personal development planning (PDP) meetings and used to guide future learning. An example of this process in practice follows.

## 10.9   A Personal Audit of NMP Practice

As stated, the generalist nature of the HAN ANP role results in NMP core formularies that include a diverse range of drugs across multiple specialties. This is in comparison with ANPs working within specialist areas who prescribe from small, well-defined formularies. For me, the scope of HAN practice brought with it an important question—how do you decide which drugs are most applicable to your role?

In preparation for NMP practice, I carried out a small audit using a convenience sample ($n = 32$) of the first patients I assessed as part of the competency framework for the NMP module. I recorded the drugs I wrote up using the existing PGD model, plus the medical prescriptions that were required for each patient. These figures were used to develop my initial core personal formulary as they provided an indication of the drugs I would be most likely to require competence in prescribing.

During my first year of prescribing practice, I recorded every prescription I wrote ($n = 207$). At the end of the year, I collated the data and, where applicable ($n = 150$), compared the data with figures from my first audit. The following table indicates three things: a comparison between PGD and NMP, a comparison between medical and NMP and the difference between the prescriptions required at the front door (FD) and in the ward areas (WA) (Table 10.1).

Whilst these figures are not directly comparable in terms of numbers, they give an indication of the difference between

**Table 10.1** Indicating a comparison between PGD and NMP, a comparison between medical and NMP and the difference between the prescriptions required at the front door (FD) and in the ward areas (WA)

| Prescription | PGD (FD) | NMP (WA) | Prescription | Medical prescription (FD) | NMP (WA) |
|---|---|---|---|---|---|
| Intravenous fluids | 19 | 91 | Antibiotics | 15 | 12 |
| Analgesia | 4 | 22 | LMWH | 1 | 0 |
| Nebulisers | 3 | 9 | Insulin/dextrose | 4 | 2 |
| Anti-emetics | 1 | 12 | Furosemide | 4 | 2 |
| No prescription indicated | 5 | Not recorded | Discontinue | 8 | Not recorded |

prescribing for newly admitted patients and those already established on treatment. During the NMP module, I spent the majority of my shifts clerking acute medical admissions. Now, as a NMP, I work mainly in an allocated group of wards comprising medicine of the elderly, acute stroke, respiratory and cardiothoracics. My core formulary has had to expand considerably, impacting on the time and effort required to achieve and maintain my prescribing competence.

I have also started recording when I decide not to prescribe a medication, which medication was requested, as well as whether the decision not to prescribe was discussed and agreed with the patient. Firstly, I am trying to evaluate my own practice from the perspective of meeting best practice standards for shared care. Secondly, I am trying to assess my practice in terms of safe prescribing. Lastly, I am evaluating whether I need to provide support and education to nursing staff that request prescriptions I decide are not appropriate.

Whilst the data I have collated so far is of a small volume, it indicates that sedation and antibiotics are the two medication groups where a prescription is most often requested yet not written.

## 10.10 Personal CPD Strategy

To meet the needs of CPD, I am currently in process of developing a learning set for those who non-medically prescribe within the HAN team. My main aims for doing this are:

- To provide a forum for discussion, peer reflection and support
- To identify learning needs arising from prescribing in specific situations taken directly from our practice
- To arrange teaching to address those needs

The main barrier to this initiative is time. In a team covering three separate sites, who work nightshift and (on one site only) weekend dayshift, plus building in factors such as family commitments and commuting distances, when is the best time to hold a meeting? This issue is one that has yet to be resolved. One possible solution involves using the shared hard drive to post relevant articles, links and feedback from personal learning such as attendance at conferences and teaching in the clinical area.

As NMP becomes more embedded in NHS culture, there are an increasing number of conferences and online learning resources available. Until now, for ANPs working in the acute setting, one major concern was the focus on NMP in the community setting. Whilst this added to a general understanding of the potential applications for NMP, it bore no relationship to the development needs of an ANP working in an acute environment. This is starting to change with the inclusion of NMP experiences of prescribing in acute practice, but there is a need for targeted educational opportunities for the acute sector.

## 10.11   Conclusion

Driven by the demands of a dynamic healthcare service that is constantly evolving to meet patient demands and expectations, and in an environment of scarce resources and rapidly changing healthcare options, there is a need for experienced ANPs who non-medically prescribe to deliver prompt, effective, safe patient care. On a personal level, NMP brings an added dimension to the care we provide as ANPs as we can deliver a service that minimises potential delays to treatment.

It is not possible for an ANP to be an expert in all specialties in the acute setting. Decision support tools, best practice guidelines and the opportunity to access the expertise of fellow HAN team members are essential components of safe and effective NMP practice. Effective communication and the documentation of clear escalation plans promotes seamless care between day and night teams.

The holistic nature of nursing and strong traditional skills of social interaction with patients marries well with new strategies for shared care in relation to treatment decisions and medication choices. For, at the end of the day, a prescribing decision is the result of a contract between a healthcare professional and a patient.

Access to Internet and email is required to facilitate the dissemination of best practice guidelines, safety alerts and for information on forthcoming CPD opportunities. Above all, NMP requires commitment from healthcare professionals, parent organisations and educational institutions to support this development in the advanced practice role.

## References

Arrigo M, Bettex D, Rudiger A (2014) Management of atrial fibrillation in critically ill patients. Crit Care Res Pract. Available via https://www.ncbi.nlm.nih.gov/pmc/articles/PMC3914350/. Accessed 25 Dec 2016

Colligan C, Sneddon J, Bayne G et al, on behalf of the Scottish Antimicrobial Prescribing Group (2015) Six years of a national antimicrobial stewardship programme in Scotland: where are we now? Antimicrob Resist Infect. Control 4:28. Available via http://aricjournal.biomedcentral.com/articles/10.1186/s13756-015-0068-1. Accessed 25 Dec 2016

National Institute for Health and Care Excellence (NICE) (2010) Delirium: prevention, diagnosis and management. NICE guidelines [CG103]. Available via https://www.nice.org.uk/guidance/cg103/chapter/1-Guidance. Accessed 25 Dec 2016

Nursing and Midwifery Council (NMC) (2006) Standards of proficiency for nurse and midwife prescribers. NMC. Available via https://www.nmc.org.uk/standards/additional-standards/standards-of-proficiency-for-nurse-and-midwife-prescribers/. Accessed 14 June 2017

Nursing and Midwifery Council (NMC) (2008) Circular 16 Remote assessment and prescribing. NMC. Available via https://www.nmc.org.uk/globalassets/sitedocuments/circulars/2008circulars/nmc-circular-16_2008.pdf. Accessed 14 June 2017

Nursing and Midwifery Council (NMC) (2015) The code: professional standards of practice for nurses and midwives. NMC [Online]. Available via https://www.nmc.org.uk/standards/code/. Accessed 14 June 2017

Scottish Government (2007) Better health better care action plan. Scottish Government. Available via http://www.gov.scot/Publications/2007/12/11103453/0. Accessed 14 June 2017

Scottish Government (2009) An evaluation of the expansion of nurse prescribing in Scotland. Scottish Government. Available via http://www.gov.scot/Publications/2009/09/24131739/0. Accessed 14 June 2017

The BMJ Group (2016, Aug) Management of hyperkalemia section 9.2.1.1 British National Formulary. Available via http://www.evidence.nhs.uk/formulary/bnf/current/9-nutrition-and-blood/92-fluids-and-electrolytes/921-oral-preparations-for-fluid-and-electrolyte-imbalance/9211-oral-potassium/management-of-hyperkalaemia. Accessed 25 Dec 2016

The National Prescribing Centre (NPC) (2012) A single competency framework for all prescribers. NPC [Online] Available at: https://www.associationforprescribers.org.uk/images/Single_Competency_Framework.pdf. Accessed 14 June 2017

# Chapter 11
# Non-medical Prescribers Within Substance Misuse Services

Hazel Roberts

**Abstract** Non-medical prescribers (NMPs) are more easily understood as prescribers who are not doctors or dentists. Within substance misuse settings, they have been functioning effectively since the non-medical independent/supplementary prescribing initiative emerged in the UK in 2006. At this time, capability to prescribe extended to make it more attractive in substance misuse service provision. Since then, within the wider context of public health drivers, NMPs in substance misuse are proven to be safe and cost-effective and to improve accessibility to medicines.

**Keywords** Substance misuse • Public health • National Treatment Agency • Supplementary prescribing • Clinical management plan • Alcohol dependence • Polypharmacy • Comorbidities • Recovery

H. Roberts
Manager and Non Medical Prescriber, Livewell South West, 200 Mount Gould Road, Plymouth, Devon, PL4 7PY, UK
e-mail: hazelroberts@nhs.net

© Springer International Publishing AG 2017
P.M. Franklin (ed.), *Non-medical Prescribing in the United Kingdom*,
DOI 10.1007/978-3-319-53324-7_11

## 11.1 Moving Forward with Ambition

The early NMP implementation focus within a public health setting was on increased access to medicines and increased responsiveness of prescribing with a hard to reach population of service users, offering empowerment and improving patient choice (DOH 2004, 2006a, 2008). Indeed cost was an important driver in the early days of NMPs in substance misuse delivery, but so too was utilising more effectively an experienced nursing workforce allowing full scope of their competencies and confidences and expanding their skills (Gossop et al. 1998a, b). Carey and Stenner (2011) describe the more relevant issues of maximising resources in a financially stretched NHS. This has undoubtedly become a primary driver for NMPs in substance misuse and progressively more so in addition to delivering high-quality care and improvements under the Department of Health's 2011 QIPP initiative (Institute for Healthcare Improvement 2011).

Despite some early interest by senior and experienced nurses in the field, prior to 2006, there were few advantages of being a substance misuse NMP because the formulary was limited. The predominant need for prescribing in substance misuse services that could be seen to improve access to medicines and fill gaps within primary care essentially was to prescribe controlled drugs within opiate substitution therapy (OST), and this still sat outside the law with significant restrictions. Despite key drivers within the service such as Her Majesty's Government's 1998 10-year drug strategy, Tackling Drugs to Build a Better Britain, the DOH 2000 NHS Plan, DOH 2004 Standards for Better Health and (DOH 2006b) Improving Patients' Access to Medicines, all we could do was watchful waiting to see how NMP developments unfolded for nurses in the field.

From 2006 onwards, the opportunity for nurses and midwives to train as both independent and supplementary prescribers (NMC 2006) meant that there were some NMP opportunities within alcohol treatment. Essentially nurse independent prescribers were able to prescribe detoxification medicines and medicines to support and promote alcohol abstinence, but these were considered to offer limited value where funding was provided predominantly for opiate and crack cocaine users remaining in established treatment for 12 weeks plus (Healthcare Commission/NTA 2006; DOH 2007; NTA 2007). Regardless of this slight progression, there remained limited prescribing parameters until the legislation changed in 2012 when amendments were made to the misuse of drugs regulations.

Despite the majority of the NMPs in substance misuse being nurses, pharmacists since 2003 have become the second largest group of professionals to become NMPs. There is a growing cohort of competent and ambitious pharmacist NMPs in the substance misuse field within community pharmacy, primary and secondary care and inpatient settings (which includes prisons). These pharmacists alongside their nursing counterparts are committed to the delivery of support across a range of practice areas. Pay grades and banding of nurses are from band 5 or equivalent in voluntary sector to band 8B for clinical nurse specialists and for some substance misuse pharmacists who are NMPs and clinical leads (Mundt-Leach 2012).

NMPs now operate in a range of settings working for a range of employers far from the conventional NHS provision. This now includes voluntary sector, charities, community interest companies (CICs), prison healthcare and private practices. Themes of delivery in substance misuse services where NMPs provide pivotal roles include the overarching wellbeing of adults within substance misuse services, their affected children, young people and families, prison communities, homelessness populations, street triage and roles within the criminal justice system broadly, pregnancy and end of life care.

Non-medical prescribers in substance misuse serve to promote, improve and enhance the health, safety and wellbeing of people who use substances in harmful and challenging ways and who may need a clinical, prescribed treatment intervention alongside psychosocial interventions as part of a recovery plan (DOH 1999; NTA 2005; Strang 2012; PHE 2014).

NMPs in substance misuse have had a tentative start in life compared to other NMPs across healthcare. This difficult birth and frustrating adolescence in the field marred by some scepticism and, one could argue, well-informed mistrust of a shifting culture led to much delay in realising the true potential of NMPs in substance misuse.

The DoH 1999 Drug Misuse and dependence UK guidelines on clinical management ("The Orange Book" to those in the trade) made mention, briefly, of the future role of nurses in prescribing. However, predominantly, the focus of this perceived bible at the time, in terms of guiding safe, effective practice in the field, was for doctors and doctors alone. In fact its central focus was guiding a range of medics in a range of settings to work to a set of standards whether they were generalist, generalist specialist or specialist. The notion of specialist and competencies required to be assigned that title could, however, be argued as relevant today with regard to NMPs at different levels of experience and operating in a range of settings.

The National Treatment Agency (NTA) for Substance Misuse services (a specialist and dedicated authority within the NHS) was established in 2001. It focused on reducing the harms to individuals, families and communities and ensuring quality and effectiveness whilst doubling the number of service users in effective treatment in the decade from 1998 to 2008 and increasing those successfully completing treatment or effectively continuing within it year over year. The NTA needed services to increase flexibility of resources to expand and ensure equitable, accessible, high-quality prescribing opportunities whilst reducing inequalities in health to service users and improving patient outcomes and workforce capabilities (Her Majesty's Government 1998). However, despite the above, managers and organisations alike had very little strategic vision or workforce plans for

NMPs in substance misuse settings, only reliant on the Department of Health or the National Treatment Agency for Substance Misuse guidance, where talk of efficiencies in the systems with regards to access to medicines appeared seductive but rarely if ever drew on the opportunities in substance misuse for NMPs specifically until 2006/2007.

As nurses existed around the substance misuse sector, this seemed like an opportunity for services to explore NMP possibilities to achieve the NTA more ambitious aims. It took some significant convincing within the system that these NMPs would be safe, competent and appropriately trained to the necessary level and would not increase prescribing costs or, indeed, increase risks to patients (Norman et al. 2010). An even then echo of the phrase "within the scope of professional competence" was representative of high levels of scrutiny both perceived and actual. The NTA stated in 2006 that nurse prescribing in substance misuse had the potential to significantly improve service delivery by ensuring the accessible supply of medication (NTA 2006) but did not at this time guide commissioners and organisations in any way as to how that would become a reality. Some early localised NMP strategies within substance misuse from 2006 onwards stated that a newly qualified NMP, regardless of area of clinical expertise, competence or time served, must prescribe within a supplementary framework using a clinical management plan (CMP) with supervision for a period of 6 months minimum or increasing to 1 year in some regions of England. This probationary period (which in the field of substance misuse had and still has, to an extent, particular value) gave newly qualified NMPs huge opportunity to gain confidence and develop their skills and in fact has led to some of the best medicine care plans that I have seen in practice.

In the early years of NMPs in substance misuse, many caveats as to the appropriate complexity of service users that they could be assigned to as supplementary prescribers had to be addressed. These were established in different areas of the UK locally.

Initially limitations around prescribing pathways were written into some local policies or prescribing frameworks, but this was not a national driver or a standardised process. Before the service users could be managed through the CMP process, they essentially first had to agree. Then they needed to be diagnosed by a doctor independent prescriber (medic). Following this a CMP that is individual to the service user would be written and agreed by a medical doctor independent prescriber, nurse supplementary prescriber and service user (DOH 2005).

NMPs, in the early days of using CMPs, were required to introduce themselves clearly as not being doctors and to record this conversation as being understood by service users as well as ensuring a quality explanation of what the CMP meant in real terms to the service user. The NMP had to be accountable and transparent within the scope of the supplementary prescribing contract and needed to avoid service user confusion and manage or contain service user expectation.

Focus of and emphasis on service delivery for the NMP agenda in the mid-2000s was all about reducing waiting times into treatment and increasing accessibility in primary care (The Effectiveness Review DOH 1996). There was a focus on shared care with primary care and specialist substance misuse services in partnership (DOH 1995, 1999, 2006a and 2006b; Gerada and Farrell 1998; Gerada and Tighe 1999). This was at a time when funding and the success of the work were shrouded in an access and retention framework with harm reduction and stabilisation language and practice being firmly on the menu (DOH 1999; NTA 2006). What this meant in essence was to get service users into treatment quickly (within 21 days of referral), to get them into some prescribed opiate substitution therapy (OST) within a very short time frame and to keep them in stabilisation beyond 12 weeks whilst encouraging a solid harm reduction model (DOH 1999, 2007). Services got paid for the amount of opiate and crack cocaine service users in treatment and for keeping them in treatment and were benchmarked nationally through reporting to NTA through the National Drug Treatment Monitoring System (NDTMs 2005).

Despite the NMP legislation in 2006 enabling NMPs more broadly to prescribe a range of drugs within the full *British National Formulary* (BNF), not only were controlled drugs off limits legally, but also the NTA 2007 stated that no NMP was expected to, and should not, prescribe from the full range of drugs listed in the BNF. The NTA 2007 document (the first in substance misuse specifically related to NMPs in the field) predominantly encouraged prescribing to a limited formulary and for specific indications (common infections, wound care, opiate withdrawal symptom management, alcohol related anti-craving medications, vitamins and emergency contraception) whilst constantly reminding NMPs only to prescribe within the competence, confidence and expertise of their practice. The focus of the supply of medicines in practice was under patient group directions and group protocols to manage minor ailments in the treatment of drug misusers (NTA 2007).

The climate of anxiety after the Shipman enquiry in 2004 (Smith 2004a and Smith 2004b) also influenced the slow development of NMPs in substance misuse. As the government commissioned a range of reports released around 2004 with recommendations for CD safer management, they had no option but to substantially strengthen governance arrangements over controlled drug management across health and social care (DOH 2006a, 2007). These included recommendations for organisations to appoint Controlled Drugs Accountable Officers (CDAOs) to make all necessary arrangement in organisations for the safe management of controlled drugs. Also, the government recommended local intelligence networks for controlled drugs (CDLINS) for sharing of information and concerns across the system. In 2007 the DOH Orange Book guidance made its first mention of the terms clinician instead of doctor throughout and made specific reference to the inclusion of non-medical prescribers, allowing us to feel reassured that we were part of the future of safe and effective prescribing within substance misuse. The last piece of guidance before the law changed to allow NMP's independent controlled drug prescribing came from the independent regulator of health and social care services in England, the Care Quality Commission (CQC) in 2010. This piece of guidance from CQC influences the way we work in substance misuse services today.

Prior to nurse independent prescribing and despite our qualification as NMPs, the legislation and the potential limitations of working only under the framework of supplementary prescribing with a CMP became frustrating, and despite various attempts to lobby and progress legislation change, this is what we had to work with. To add to practice frustration, a skilled and expert nursing workforce in substance misuse existed that could add value in a growing climate of even more for even less as cost pressures loomed large. As specialist nurses in addiction, we were confident in our skills and especially proud of our proven abilities in clinical assessment. We had already, to a certain extent, been guiding the practice of other more junior staff, medics and GPs around prescribing issues and medicines management for some time. This was often referred to as de facto prescribing, and ultimately influenced doctors prescribing practice whereby the medics merely rubber stamped by production of a prescription, the nursing recommendations and decision-making. Doctors would not themselves assess or diagnose the patients, thus creating potential patient safety concerns and patient safety compromise (Otway 2002; Carey et al. 2009; Courtenay et al. 2009).

Even with the constraints of prescribing within a supplementary framework and within the boundaries of a clinical management plan, NMPs could demonstrate quality medicines management and medicines reconciliation and review. We were skilled at early assessment, risk assessment and completing a full comprehensive healthcare assessment (NTA 2002). We were able to identify service user dependence (diagnose), identify needs and what's more identify risks whilst at the same time making suggestions as to the most appropriate and available interventions and encouraging engagement with some hard to reach service users. These skills in assessment however were not just about diagnosis of dependency for the purposes of initiating prescribing interventions but were skilled assessments within a framework of complexity. These included mental health, physical health, comorbidities including long-term conditions and complex poly-pharmacy. Of course within the parameters of the CMP, the medic would have to assess and diagnose.

As already discussed, we could prescribe independently medications other than controlled drugs for alcohol dependence or detoxification and relapse prevention medications as independent prescribers, but until 2012 controlled drug prescribing was off limits. The CMP and the title "Supplementary Prescriber" had conditions of practice attached. Although supplementary prescribers could prescribe any drugs from the BNF that were within their competence and confidence, certain distinctions were created locally in substance misuse prescribing for some areas of NMP practice in relation to assignment of cases, for example, not being able to prescribe for pregnant women, prison releases (transfer of care from prisons) or service users being released from court and service users with complex and multiple comorbidities. It was the medics (doctors) who retained this higher risk work.

NMPs, despite experience, were often encouraged to, or in some cases policies demanded that they, prescribe for people with fewer complexities and referred back to the medic independent prescriber when there were any issues of concern (these being clearly recorded in the clinical management plans). Despite eagerness and ambition to develop, early NMP positions offered limited flexibility within limited formulary options, such as prescribing options with limits to the maximum dose range and route of administration. There were also clear practice restrictions, which often included no handwritten prescriptions. Restrictions regarding the allocation of the complexity of cases were commonplace with allocation of NMPs to simple rather than complex cases being the order of the day. Non-medical prescribing was often described in a pathway where we were asked to handle more simple service user cases than our colleagues who included consultants in addiction, senior medics in secondary care addiction services and general practitioners (GPs) with special interests. However, NMPs in substance misuse were handling cases of the same level of complexity or slightly higher than GPs in primary care that had completed the level one Royal College of General Practitioners in substance misuse training (RCGP 2005). Incidentally NMPs were also attending and completing this course and similarly the RCGP training for alcohol.

In spite of increased diligence around controlled drugs (CDs) after the Shipman enquiries (2001–2004) and subsequent recommendations with regard to CD management regardless of practice setting, the law did change in 2012 enabling NMPs to prescribe controlled drugs independently, and this revolutionised the work. No longer could NMPs in substance misuse be restricted and constrained in their professional artistry since we had confidence, competence and expertise at this time and had well and truly cut our teeth with supplementary prescribing earning respect in the field from our medic and drug worker colleagues alike. A range of safeguards to the organisation, colleagues and the public which included careful selection onto training courses, quality training processes with reliable examination processes (through written exams and vivas) and robust governance frameworks enabled a flexible and safe system for providing enhanced prescribing. However, there was always the caveat that NMPs must at all times only be expected to prescribe inside their areas of competence (PHE 2014).

Five years on from 2012, we find ourselves with a very different political landscape influencing substance misuse services.

In many ways, austerity measures and managing sustainability have become the new practice based limitations rather than restrictions through legislation. Modernised systems where rapid, equitable flexible access across geographical areas and reducing waiting times have progressed (Health Care Commission and NTA 2006; DOH 2007). Of course access is still important (particularly within criminal justice settings), but from 2012 treatment retention and treatment completion have been the influential driving force with a shift of emphasis towards recovery (NTA 2010; Strang 2012; National Treatment Agency Drug Misuse and Dependence Guidance Draft 2016. Available via http://www.nta.nhs.uk/guidelines.aspx. Accessed 15th June 2017).

The NTA 2007 estimated that there were approximately 80 nurses and pharmacists working in the treatment of substance misuse who were either active prescribers, in training or contemplating training as NMPs. What's more, a 2012 mapping exercise across the UK heavily supported by the National Substance Misuse Non-Medical Prescribing Forum (NSMNMPF). Available via http://www.nmpsm.org/. Accessed 15th June 2017 established that there were at least 316 NMPs in England in various settings and with diverse prescribing roles (Mundt-Leach and Hill 2014). This demonstrates significant increase in the scope of NMP practice in substance misuse services, and it's likely that these numbers will continue to increase.

To date, NMPs operate effectively within what remains a stigmatised area of healthcare, amidst a varied and diversely skilled substance misuse staffing component and within a challenging healthcare and public health landscape. NMPs offer significant added value in the delivery of quality and effective drug treatment interventions but add much more than that. They are not only visible within the workforce and within their professional bodies but are now part of a system that drives efficiencies, shifting prescribing from the traditional domains of medicine and medic (once the preserve of our doctors who we are in admiration of and hold tremendous respect for) to a multi-professional platform (Morgan-Henshaw and Ishmael 2015).

NMPs in the field can now fully embrace the scope of practice as independent prescribers being able to assess, diagnose and treat drug and alcohol dependence (PHE 2014) and are crucial within a rapidly changing NHS. Organisational NMP strategies are now fully inclusive of the work of NMPs in the field. And since the Public Health England guidance in July 2014, organisations have greater accountability to the NMPs to offer the appropriate governance, supervision and opportunity for continuing professional development (CPD). This latest document specifically related to NMPs in substance misuse serves to guide the employing organisation and the NMP towards a strategic focus moving forward with ambition, setting standards for supervision, line management, CPD and prescribing competencies.

With the exception of highly specialised and indeed contentious medical treatments such as the prescribing of diamorphine for addiction, and some local formulary, budgetary or commissioning constraints (which will be unique across regions), substance misuse NMPs participate and lead teams within influential roles, delivering excellence and value for money and providing the comprehensive menu of interventions across all stages of treatment tiers within the field. They have wide-ranging practice and leadership roles offering opportunities to innovate, increase productivity and drive effectiveness, and there is growing evidence that non-medical prescribing makes a real difference to the care of vulnerable patients in a wider range of health and social care settings. For service users who find it difficult to engage in primary/secondary care settings, NMPs offering prompt assessment and prescribing assessments, diagnosis and prescribing reviews in flexible settings are proven to be invaluable (Carey and Stenner 2011).

The widening scope of practice has occurred through practice confidence and competence, public confidence and indeed service user's confidence and satisfaction. In addition to that however (invariably a symptom of austerity), added demands on services and organisations to offer best value for money have revisited the cheaper doctor argument. Most organisations that employ NMPs now have to have NMP leads, strategies and workforce plans (DOH 2006b) which include a widening scope of NMP practice, and substance misuse is no different. Most senior nurses in the substance misuse field are encouraged, if eligible, to consider NMP as an essential development to their role.

Since gaining respect and a level, in some areas, of admiration, we are asked to deliver sessions, as part of training courses, and conferences and indeed offer supervision to our medic colleagues. All prescribers now focus on collaboration and cooperation and coproduction at all levels, aided by a single prescriber competency framework (2016), which does not differentiate the profession of the prescriber. What emerges therefore from this lack of differentiation is, prescribers working together, learning together and developing their art together (National Prescribing Centre Single Competency Framework 2012 and more recently the Royal Pharmaceutical Society prescribing Competency Framework for All Prescribers 2016). Now prescribers are ultimately singing from the same hymn sheet in terms of adherence to the same competencies to evidence safe and effective prescribing practice. It is undoubtedly relevant to inspire integrated high-quality prescribing resources, which are much needed and will continue to improve the patient experience, reduce risks and ultimately save money.

With recovery models and theories having been such an important development in the field since 2007 (NTA 2007 guidelines and current revision of the orange book guidelines), it's time, also, for NMPs in the field to stretch their wings, having a larger span of influence and growing credibility in the treatment system especially the recovery focus. Strang (2012) reviewed the substance misuse treatment system and made mention of the criticism that service users were being merely parked in prescribed interventions in treatment, and NMPs saw that they have as part of a wider multidisciplinary team approach a wider part to play. With the previous focus often but not exclusively on pharmacological interventions, other allied healthcare professionals/drug and alcohol workers could concentrate on psychosocial interventions and optimising the service user's recovery capital in a series of domains. One could argue that the very presence of the first NMPs perpetuated an awareness of the above and greater sense of value for them.

Having gained mutual respect and parity of esteem amongst our prescribing colleagues, the increased benefit to the service user is clearly identifiable and evidenced (Dowden 2016). But what does this mean for us as treatment services are encouraged towards another new phase of change, delivering truly global recovery outcomes? What can happen in terms of NMP innovation?

Current practice includes nurses, pharmacists, medics and allied health professionals working together following quality prescribing frameworks, and linking their governance and their education wherever possible. This is strongly supported and evidenced through the NMPSMF (www.nmpsm.org). This forum delivers a series of national and local events specific to the needs of non-medical prescribers in the field in relation to CPD, information sharing, dissemination of good practice and looking at complex cases or practice dilemmas and debating joint/shared care delivery issues.

No longer are services seeing year on year investments in substance misuse. Since the Health and Social Care Act 2012, the removal of ring-fenced money to the field, making the services work harder to evidence outcomes and find best value recovery solutions, is an ongoing challenge to sustainability as we sit alongside other public health areas vying for the investment. Key NHS England 5 Year Forward View 2016 plans that affect GPs and primary care, mental health and the NHS broadly (NHS England 2014; Public Health England 2014; Mental Health Taskforce to the NHS in England 2014) offer challenges within the system not just about sustainability but proffers questions that have changed from "what is the matter with you?" to "what matters to you?", a subtle linguistic change but an important practice influencer. Subtle organisational linguistic changes, such as from "patients" to "people", "care settings" to "places of care" and "organisations" to "networks of care", prompt changes to the paradigm of the doctor/nurse/patient/service user relationship and the power balance within modern healthcare. They ask us to think differently about our work.

Thirty years ago, the idea that nurses with a specialist practice qualification could prescribe dressings and topical treatments in district nursing settings is a far cry from where we find ourselves today. The stage has been set for the current and future developments in the field of substance misuse for NMPs, and it is exciting indeed. We can now prescribe within our scope of practice and as nurse independent prescribers licensed, unlicensed and for uses outside of product licence (off label) medications. What's more and as a result of changes in 2012 to the misuse of drugs regulations, most controlled drugs listed in schedules 2–5 where it is clinically appropriate and within our professional competence (except for cocaine, diamorphine and dipipanone for the treatment of addiction) Available via https://www.rcn.org.uk/get-help/rcn-advice/nurse-prescribing#Nurse%20independent%20prescribers%20and%20controlled%20drugs%20-%20changes%20to%20

the%20Misuse%20of%20Drugs%20Regulations. Accessed 27th
Dec 2016.

We are confident to rise to the challenges of future service
provision as drug trends and changes in public health policy and
practice influence the field.

# References

Care Quality Commission (2010) Guidance about compliance: essential
standards of quality and safety. Available via http://www.cqc.org.uk/
sites/default/files/documents/guidance_about_compliance_summary.
pdf. Accessed 27 Dec 2016

Carey N, Stenner K (2011) Does non-medical prescribing make a difference? Nurs Times 107(26):14–16

Carey N et al (2009) Prescription writing for patients with diabetes: compliance with good practice. Nurse Prescr 7(10):464–468

Courtenay M et al (2009) Nurse prescriber patient consultations: a case
study in dermatology. J Adv Nurs 65(6):1207–1217

Department of Health (1995) Reviewed shared care arrangements for drug
misusers. DOH, London. (Executive letter); EL (95)114

Department of Health (1996) Task force to review services for drug misusers: report of an independent review of drug treatment services in
England. Department of Health, London

Department of Health (1999) Drug misuse and dependence: UK guidelines
on clinical management. Department of Health (England), London, The
Scottish Office Department of Health, Welsh Office and Department of
Health and Social Services, Northern Ireland, The Stationery Office

Department of Health (2000) The NHS plan: a plan for investment, a plan
for reform. The Stationery Office, London

Department of Health (2004) Standards for better health. The Stationery
Office, London

Department of Health (2005) Supplementary prescribing by nurses, pharmacists, chiropodists/podiatrists, physiotherapists and radiographers
within the NHS in England: a guide for implementation. The Stationery
Office, London

Department of Health (2006a) Safer management of controlled drugs: (1)
guidance on strengthened governance arrangements, March 2006,
updated January. Available via http://webarchive.nationalarchives.gov.

uk/20130107105354/http://www.dh.gov.uk/en/Publicationsandstatistics/ Publications/PublicationsPolicyAndGuidance/DH_064460. Accessed 27 Dec 2016

Department of Health (2006b) Improving patients access to medicines. The Stationery Office, London

Department of Health Safer management of controlled drugs: (1) guidance on strengthened governance arrangements, March 2006d, updated January 2007. Available via http://webarchive.nationalarchives.gov. uk/20130107105354/http://www.dh.gov.uk/en/Publicationsandstatistics/ Publications/PublicationsPolicyAndGuidance/DH_064460. Accessed 27 Dec 2016

Department of Health (2008) Making connections: using healthcare professionals as prescribers to deliver organisational improvements. The Stationery Office, London

Department of Health (2011) Quality, innovation, productivity and prevention (QIPP) 2011. Available via http://webarchive.nationalarchives.gov. uk/20130107105354/http://dh.gov.uk/health/category/policy-areas/nhs/ quality/qipp/. Accessed 27 Dec 2016

Department of Health (England) and the Devolved Administrations (2007) Drug misuse and dependence: UK guidelines on clinical management

Department of Health (England), London The Scottish government, welsh assembly government and Northern Ireland executive. Available via http://www.nta.nhs.uk/uploads/clinical_guidelines_2007.pdf. Accessed 27 Dec 2016

Department of Health England (2016) Drug misuse and dependence: UK guidelines on clinical management. Consultation on updated draft 2016 (2016) Available via http://www.nta.nhs.uk/uploads/cg-2016-consultation-draft.pdf. Accessed 7 July 2017

Dowden A (2016) The expanding role of nurse prescribers. Prescriber 27(6):1–7

Gerada C, Farrell M (1998) Shared care. In: Robertson JR (ed) Management of drug users in the community: a practical handbook. Arnold, London, pp 328–352

Gerada C, Tighe J (1999) A review of shared care protocols for the treatment of problem drug use in England, Scotland and Wales. Br J Gener Pract 49(439):125–126

Gossop M, Marsden J, Stewart D (1998a) NTORS at one year: changes in substance use, health and criminal behaviors one year after intake. Department of Health, London

Gossop M, Marsden J, Stewart D et al (1998b) Substance use, health and social problems of clients at 54 drug agencies: intake data from the national treatment outcome research study (NTORS). Br J Psychiatry 173:166–171

Healthcare Commission (NHS) and National Treatment Agency for substance misuse (2006) Improving services for substance misuse. A Joint Review. Commission for Healthcare Audit and Inspection. Available via http://www.nta.nhs.uk/uploads/joint_reviewfull_report_0506.pdf. Accessed 27 Dec 2016

Her Majesty's Government (1998) Tackling drugs to build a better Britain: the government's ten-year strategy for tackling drug misuse. The Stationery Office, London (CM 3945)

Institute for Healthcare Improvement (2011) Impacting Cost and Quality Program 2011. Available via http://www.ihi.org/Engage/Initiatives/Completed/IMPACTingCostQuality/Documents/Impactingbrochure2011final.pdf. Accessed 15 June 2017

Latter S, Blenkinsopp A, Smith A et al (2010) Evaluation of nurse and pharmacist prescribing. Executive summary. Department of Health, London

Mental Health Taskforce to the NHS England (2016) The five-year forward view for mental health. NHS England. Available via https://www.england.nhs.uk/mental-health/taskforce/. Accessed 15 June 2017

Morgan-Henshaw P, Ishmael A (2015) Preceptor programmes in mental health. Nurse Prescr 13(3):146–147

Mundt-Leach R (2012) Non-medical prescribing by specialist addictions nurses. Mental Health Pract 16(3):24–27

Mundt-Leach R, Hill D (2014) Non-medical prescribing in substance misuse services in England and Scotland: a mapping exercise. J Mental Health Pract 17(9):28–35

Mundt-Leach R blog. Available via SMMGP. org.uk/blog/?p=24. Accessed 24 Mar 2016

National Institute for Health and Clinical Excellence and The National Prescribing Centre (2012) A single competency framework for all prescribers. Available via https://www.associationforprescribers.org.uk/images/Single_Competency_Framework.pdf. Accessed 14 June 2017

National Treatment Agency (2002) Models of care for treatment of adult drug misusers. Available via http://www.nta.nhs.uk/uploads/nta_modelsofcare2_2002_moc2.pdf. Accessed 15 June 2017

National Treatment Agency and Department of Health (2005) statistics for the national drug treatment monitoring system (NDTMS). Available via http://www.nta.nhs.uk/statistics.aspx. Accessed 27 Dec 2016

National Treatment Agency for Substance Misuse (NHS) (2007) Non-medical prescribing, patient group directions and minor ailment schemes in the treatment of drug misusers. Available via www.nta.nhs.uk/nmp-in-the-management-of-substance-misuse-2014.aspx. Accessed 27 Dec 2016

NHS (2014) Five year forward plan. Available via https://www.england.nhs.uk/wp-content/uploads/2014/10/5yfv-web.pdf. Accessed 27 Dec 2016

NICE (2007a) Drug misuse: psychosocial interventions. NICE clinical guidelines 51. National Institute for Health and Clinical Excellence, London

NICE (2007b) Drug misuse: opioid detoxification. NICE clinical guideline 52. National Institute for Health and Clinical Excellence, London

NICE (2007c) Methadone and buprenorphine for the management of opioid dependence. NICE technology appraisal guidance 114. National Institute for Health and Clinical Excellence, London

Norman IJ et al (2010) A comparison of the clinical effectiveness and costs of mental health nurse supplementary prescribing and independent medical prescribing a post-test control group study. BMC Health Serv Res 10(4):1–9

Nursing and Midwifery Council (2006) Standards of proficiency for nurse and midwife prescribers. NMC, London

Otway C (2002) The development needs of nurse prescribers. Nurs Stand 16(18):33–38

Public Health England (2014) Non-medical prescribing in the management of substance misuse. National Substance Misuse Non-Medical Prescribing Forum. Available via http://www.nta.nhs.uk/uploads/nmp-in-the-management-of-substance-misuse.pdf Accessed 7 July 2017)

Public Health England (2014) Non-medical prescribing in the management of substance misuse. PHE, London

RCGP Royal College of General Practitioners (n.d.) Available via www.rcgp.org.uk/substance-misuse. Accessed 27 Dec 2016

Royal College of Psychiatrists and Royal College of General Practitioners (2005) Roles and responsibilities of doctors in the provision of treatment for drug and alcohol misusers. Council report CR131. Royal College of Psychiatrists and General Practitioners, London

Royal College of Nursing (n.d.) Nurse prescribing. Available via https://www.rcn.org.uk/get-help/rcn-advice/nurse-prescribing#Nurse%20independent%20prescribers%20and%20controlled%20drugs%20-%20changes%20to%20the%20Misuse%20of%20Drugs%20Regulations. Accessed 27 Dec 2016

Royal Pharmaceutical Society (2016) A competency framework for all prescribers. The Royal Pharmaceutical Society, London

Smith, DJ (2004a) Fourth report of the shipman inquiry: the regulation of controlled drugs in the community. Available via http://webarchive.nationalarchives.gov.uk/20090808154959/http://www.the-shipman-inquiry.org.uk/fourthreport.asp. Accessed 27 Dec 2016

Smith, DJ (2004b) Fifth report of the shipman inquiry: safeguarding patients: lessons from the past—proposals for the future. Available via http://www.shipman-inquiry.org.uk/fifthreport.asp. Accessed 27 Dec 2016

Strang J (2012) Medications in recovery: re-orientating drug dependence treatment. National Treatment Agency, London

# Chapter 12
# Non-medical Prescribing in Palliative and End-of-Life Care (EOLC)

**Emma Sweeney**

**Abstract**   The one certainty in life is that we will all die, and the only unpredictable factor is how and where. UK nurses have the authority to prescribe after completion of a recognised accredited prescribing course through a UK university. However, a relatively small number of nurses train as prescribers and many who qualify do not utilise their skills on a regular basis. Clinical Nurse Specialists (CNS) in palliative care are rightly reluctant to prescribe relevant drugs without the appropriate support or training and lack of support and acceptance by the medical team. Commonly prescribed drugs such as opioids, anti-emetics, anti-secretory drugs, antipsychotic agents and mouth care products can significantly enhance the role of the CNS in palliative care and the support and care provided for our dying patients.

E. Sweeney
University Hospital Southampton NHS Foundation Trust,
Tremona Road, Southampton, Hampshire SO16 6YD, UK
e-mail: Emma.Sweeney@colchesterhospital.nhs.uk

© Springer International Publishing AG 2017                      215
P.M. Franklin (ed.), *Non-medical Prescribing in the United Kingdom*,
DOI 10.1007/978-3-319-53324-7_12

**Keywords** Clinical Nurse Specialists • Palliative
care • End-of-life care (EOLC) • Anticipatory medicines
• Pain management • Hospice • Community • Training and
support

## 12.1 Introduction: Background to Palliative and EOLC

Palliative care will always be a necessity, as people will always
die. The way in which care and services are delivered will have
an impact on those affected by death as well as those working
within palliative care. People who are dying, their loved ones
and families will have wishes, preferences of place of care and
death that should always be considered providing individualised
care to everyone. There will be a percentage of those that are
dying that will experience symptoms commonly associated in
the last days of life which include pain, nausea and vomiting,
agitation and excess chest secretions of which nurses who are
non-medical prescribers will be working with patients and their
families to minimise or if successful completely control.

The inevitably of death presents challenges in that 99% of
deaths are adults aged 18+ with most of the deaths occurring in
those 65 and over. 500,000 million people die in England each
year. A large majority of deaths in the twenty-first century follow a period of chronic ill health such as heart disease, cancer,
stroke, chronic respiratory disease, neurological disease or
dementia. 58% of deaths occur in acute hospital Trusts. One of
the key points raised for most people when end-of-life care is
approaching and discussed is that they have a good death which
incorporates being without pain and other symptoms. Many
people experience unnecessary pain and other symptoms; these
can lead to distress both emotionally and physically and lead to
the lack of dignity and respect (DH 2008).

The National End of Life Care Strategy (DH 2008) was developed with over 300 stakeholders to develop a care pathway, which would include the delivery of high-quality services in all locations and management of the last days of life. The document sets out the following key point: ensuring health and social care staff at all levels have the necessary knowledge, skills and attitudes related to care for the dying as this will be critical to the success of improving EOLC. The strategy also sets out that it means for patients this includes high-quality care and support during the last days of life, stating that this should be planned and well-coordinated. Within the document, it is recognised that acute hospitals are the most common place of death, and it is widely recognised that:

- We do not talk openly about death and dying.
- It is difficult to initiate discussions for those approaching the end of their life.
- There are difficulties in eliciting people's needs and preferences.
- Care and support should be 24 h a day.
- There can be inadequate training of health and social care staff, resulting in gaps in care and inappropriate care delivery.

It is also recognised that people experience unnecessary physical and psychological suffering if the above points are not acted on appropriately.

In total between June 2004 and July 2006 across all NHS organisations, there were a total of 16,000 complaints of which no less than 54% related to EOLC in some way (DH 2008). One of the common themes that arose from the complaints was due to the lack of basic comfort, which would include a patient's symptom control management.

The nature of the condition from which people are suffering when they enter the dying phase and the variety of different presenting symptoms that they cause means that patients with similar diagnosis and symptomatology may often take different trajectories in the last days of life. It can prove difficult therefore to take a holistic approach to their management. It is noted that many people in the older age population have several coexisting health problems, which may make symptoms difficult to manage when a person is dying.

Peoples' health might also decline either rapidly, or present as a gradual decline in those that are frail with a slower progression over months and years, and these factors need to be taken into account when contributing to a symptom-free death.

The DH 2008 strategy also states that there are common requirements for workforce development in specialist palliative care. For example, training must ensure that those involved in palliative and EOLC take into account appropriate assessment of peoples' needs and that symptom control management is undertaken at all times.

Around 5500 staff work in specialist and palliative care services, and they have a vital role in providing education for staff who are not specialists. The 2008 strategy highlights that there are specific training needs for this cohort of staff and that this should be adequately resourced by employers. However, in times of financial difficulty, this can sometimes be hard to achieve. For example, in NHS organisations, funding for study leave has been significantly reduced, and funding may have to be resourced personally or by charitable organisations. This is coupled with the challenge that time to attend study leave due to pressures on organisations regarding staffing may also prohibit staff from having study leave granted or it being cancelled at short notice.

The Ambitions of Palliative and End Of Life Care: A national framework for local action 2015–2020—National Palliative and End of life care partnership (National Palliative and End of Life Partnership 2015) set out six ambitions, one of which is maximising comfort and well-being and should encompass the following statement for patients:

My care is regularly reviewed and every effort is made for me to
have the support, care and treatment that might be needed  to help
me to be as comfortable and as free from distress as possible. p. 11

The ambitions state that there are five key priorities for the
person who is dying of which one is directly related to symptom
control management, highlighting that professionals need to
address and work to alleviate the causes of physical and emotional distress at the end of life.

## 12.2  What the Literature Says

Ziegler et al. (2015) highlight that the United Kingdom (UK) is
considered to be the world leader in nurse prescribing; no other
country have the same extended non-medical prescribing rights.
However, research into the benefits has yet to match the number
of extended roles such as non-medical prescribers in complex
areas such as palliative care.

Culshaw et al. (2013) report that the use of 'off label' drugs
(drugs used outside of the specifications for which they are
licensed) is widespread in palliative care. This is a legal practice; however, non-medical prescribers should be aware that
specific guidelines should be followed as set out by the NMC
2006 and 2015. A survey was carried out in 2013 of prescribers
including non-medical prescribers in palliative care to see how
they adhered to the guidance. The responses noted that there
were few organisations stating that they had a policy setting out
the expectations and information relating to off label drugs. This
could therefore set out a challenge when prescribing for those
with complex symptoms as the result of the dying process.

Quinn and Lawrie (2010) state that NMP has been at the
centre of government policy in the UK and is a vehicle to
improve patient care and highlight the positives for Clinical
Nurse Specialists (CNSs) working in palliative care. They high-

light the need for guidance to support providers and that it is essential to promote confidence in the scope of prescribing. As CNSs often work autonomously, it is important to provide mentoring following the qualification as a non-medical prescriber.

Wilson et al. (2015) state that the UK had a way of improving EOLC, which included the introduction of anticipatory medication. These medicines are there just in case symptoms arise for those who are dying. Nurses have the responsibility to decide when the patient requires anticipatory medications. Anticipatory medications enable patients to be comforted and settled with gradual relief of symptoms at the lowest dose possible. Anticipatory medications are designed to respond quickly to individual needs and within the community setting aiming to avoid hospital admissions and allow people to die in their preferred place of death if it is not the hospital environment.

Lennan (2014) states that independent prescribers including those in palliative care require consistent regulatory guidance to support them in the care provision for those who are at the end of their life. Often patients who are entering the dying phase of their life have multiple symptoms and coupled with the complexities of organ failure can pose the ultimate challenge in the world of non-medical prescribing. Therefore, those professionals who prescribe in the specialism of palliative care need the access to guidance and support from those who currently prescribe to have the forum to discuss how patient's symptoms can be managed. For example, ketamine can be prescribed for complex pain and is licensed for use in palliative care; however, it is not commonly used as a first- or second-line analgesic.

Stenner et al. (2012) state that indications are that nurses can improve treatment and access to pain medications when they prescribe. However, we must consider the training needs of these nurses. Continuing to invest in this support will allow them to have the confidence and competence to prescribe a wider range of medication which is essential in palliative and end-of-life care. Other symptoms associated with those who are dying, such as the symptoms associated with constipation, can cause patients physical discomfort and psychological distress (Andrews and Morgan 2012). Palliative care nurses are also highly skilled in managing other symptoms related to dying such as nausea and sickness, agitation and a high volume of chest secretions. These are common symptoms associated with the dying process and commonly observed as part of the assessment of a specialist palliative care nurse. As with pain management at end of life, although there is a standardised set of recommended drugs that can be used to assist in controlling these symptoms to support people who are dying, there are some patients who require constant management and readjustment of drugs to work towards symptom control.

Webb and Gibson (2011) highlight the positive impact that non-medical prescribing has on patient and palliative care. They recognise that some palliative care services also provide a 7-day and out-of-hour service which enhances the role of the CNS enabling provision of a timely and appropriate approach to providing care for those at the end of their lives.

Creddon and O'Regan (2010) highlight that pain at the end of life is a significant symptom of anxiety and distress, which can often be debilitating and feared by those at the end of their lives. This requires expert interventions by specialist palliative care professionals as they have expert knowledge on treatments and symptoms management in order to address and manage pain appropriately. To enhance this, nurse prescribers in palliative care can address the issue of inadequate pain management by facilitating access to medication in a timelier manner.

Farrell et al. (2011) state that changes have taken place to nurses' roles, and thus their clinical responsibilities over the past decade have changed. This has led to new ways of working and in turn higher levels of nursing practice. There are prescribing benefits for both patients and nurses who strive towards more enhanced approach to multidisciplinary working. Dawson (2013) states that within adult community palliative care, there has been a drive to improve the quality of care for these patients by providing a flexible and streamlined service, one of these areas is in non-medical prescribing.

Non-medical prescribing gives patients quicker access to medicines as well as improving access to services and makes better use of health-care professional skills. Of course, nurse prescribers must work within their own levels of professional competence (NMC 2006). The implications for nurses with the above statement in mind is that this may lead to under prescribing as there can be circumstances where drugs that aren't licensed for symptom control in palliative care but may be indicated. Nurses' caution with regard to prescribing off label (otherwise known as outside of product license) is understandable; however, this could potentially have a negative impact on access to efficient symptom control, which is unacceptable.

Cole and Gillet (2015) discuss that prescribing in palliative care was an early candidate area for the extension of nurse prescribing authority but despite this has failed to meet the expectations of the prescribers. There are a low proportion of palliative care nurse specialists that possess the prescribing qualification, and little work has been done to undertake evaluation of the specialist palliative care prescribers' experience in prescribing as well as the outcome and influences to their practice with patients.

NICE guidance care of the dying adult in the last days of life (2015) guideline covers the clinical care of adults (18 years and over) who are dying during the last 2–3 days of life. It aims to improve end-of-life care for people in their last days of life by communicating respectfully and involving them, and the people important to them, in decisions and by maintaining their comfort and dignity. The guideline covers how to manage common symptoms without causing unacceptable side effects and how to maintain hydration in the last days of life.

This guideline includes recommendations on:

- Recognising when people are entering the last few days of life
- Communicating and shared decision-making
- Clinically assisted hydration
- Medicines for managing pain, breathlessness, nausea and vomiting, anxiety, delirium, agitation and noisy secretions
- Anticipatory prescribing

NICE (2004) supportive and palliative care guidance highlights that patients and families with a life limiting diagnosis should be assessed holistically. This is to ensure that their care is co-ordinated openly and sensitively and that all basic levels of symptoms control are maintained. It is documented within the report that care for our dying patients can often be suboptimal in a variety of care settings (acute hospital Trusts, a patient home and care homes) as recognition and sometimes acknowledgement of the dying patient does not often occur in a timely manner. The guidance objectives specifically state that all patients need to have a dignified death, with family and other carers adequately supporting during the process and which would incorporate symptom control and management.

The guidelines also state that within the community there is a 24 hour service of 7 days a week for those with advanced disease. This is accompanied by a set of key components of best practice in community palliative care which are that patients are regularly assessed and anticipated needs are noted, planned for and addressed; this would include the prescription of anticipatory medications. Prescriptions of anticipatory medications are a mechanism to aid the management of the common symptoms associated with the dying process such as pain, nausea and vomiting, agitation and increased chest secretions. The guidance also states that current medications are assessed and non-essential medicines are discontinued; non-medical prescribers would be able to have the autonomy to prescribe anticipatory medicines and discontinue those that are now no longer essential.

The guidance also notes that failure to recognise the dying patient whether this is due to lack of training can prevent the relevant care (including medicines management) being commenced. NICE (2004) backs this up by stating that programmes of education and training in particular relation to management have been shown to lead improvements in knowledge, attitudes and clinical behaviours of staff involved in caring for those who are dying.

## 12.3   The Role of the Clinical Nurse Specialist in Palliative Care

Clinical Nurse Specialists (CNSs) have a vital role in delivery of high-quality and compassionate care in a variety of specialisms or settings including palliative and end-of-life care. CNSs are the frontline of care and are key to improving the patient's outcomes and experiences. In the context of palliative care, outcomes will be to achieve a good death, which will include good symptom management. CNSs are often the main point of contact for patients and their loved ones/carers and through their work and working very closely with patients can contribute and often lead in shaping services that are patient centred incorporating their needs and choices. This is pertinent when working with patients with life-limiting illnesses; it is important to undertake a thorough holistic assessment, which incorporates a physical assessment (to include any symptoms changes/responses in symptomatology) as a result of pharmacotherapeutic intervention.

Contact from a CNS in palliative care can assist in increasing the quality of care provided by the National Health Service (NHS). When a patient is faced with the dying process or a non-curable diagnosis, many emotions and expectations can manifest. This can lead to heightened expectations and result in the intrinsic link between psychological and physical symptoms.

Within palliative and end-of-life care, CNSs work within acute trusts and community settings and more often than not support the same patients as they move between health-care organisations for specific time periods within their pathway. It is therefore essential that communication and collaborative working is promoted to ensure the patient and their loved ones are supported seamlessly with continuity at all times.

The role of the CNS has evolved over time to incorporate technical elements which has in some cases transformed into a practitioner working towards or at a masters' level qualification possessing specialist knowledge and skills within the area they work, and this remains the case for palliative care CNSs. Many palliative care CNSs strive to undertake an academic physical assessment and consultation module, which is essential to their role and a natural progression towards the non-medical prescribing qualification. CNSs work autonomously and as a core member of a multidisciplinary team (MDT) where they work alongside other professionals to treat and manage the health concerns of patients.

It is important to consider prescribing in palliative care that is delivered across a variety of all care settings and will be discussed in succession below.

## 12.4   Hospice

Hospices are a support provision of a caring environment that is designed to meet both the physical and emotional needs of those with non-curable illnesses. Hospice services are often made up of an inpatient unit where people come to die or, for complex symptom management and an array of community services. These can often comprise of day services for patients, support groups ranging from creative art to counselling and community facing services such as Hospice at Home where direct care can be provided to those and their families who are dying at home. Hospice staff usually specialise in the field of palliative and end-of-life care providing support to those who access their services. Patient and carer feedback on the whole is usually positive. Unfortunately many Hospice inpatient units are relatively small (i.e. number of beds) which would therefore raise the concern that some patients who are fortunate to access hospice service receive the best possible care at the end of their life; however, equity across the geographical location can be disputed. As a result, this may lead to inappropriate delays in accessing community services or admission into their local hospital. Many nurses who work within a hospice setting do not require possessing or working towards a non-medical prescribing qualification, as specialty doctors are always available. This could potentially lead to the nurses feeling deskilled within their area of practice.

## 12.5  Community

The role of the Community Palliative Care Clinical Nurse Specialist (CNS) differs from that of the acute trust CNS in that those who work within a community setting assess, monitor and review patients in their own homes. Some community palliative care teams set within a hospice setting therefore having direct access to specialist doctors can enhance the patients' and their families' experience at the end of their life.

The benefits to community CNSs in palliative care being non-medical prescribers are that there is an automatic response to the assessment undertaken by the CNS in managing their symptoms. This can have a direct positive impact to enhance the patients' pathway even when you think away from the common anticipatory prescribing in the last days of someone's life but focus on simple yet every effective treatments such as oral thrush which can be distressing for the patient who cannot maintain their own oral hygiene needs.

Conversely having specialist nurses undertaking the prescribing responsibility for patients who are dying in the community may divert responsibility from general practitioners (GPs) who are the patients' primary carer in supporting patients and their families during and following a death occurring. As GP's caseloads are increasingly busy, it is important for them to have an overall awareness of their dying patient's needs (this is usually through a monthly Gold Standards Framework (GSF) meeting), but for those who are dying, it is essential for NMPs to communicate frequently with the GP regarding symptoms and any alterations made to assist in the effect management of symptoms in the last days of life.

## 12.6    Maintaining Training: Training and Support for NMPs

The NMC Standards (2015) state that there is a standard set for education and training which accompanies the additional skill of being a non-medical prescriber. It is of imperative importance that the conduct and performance of NMPs ensure the safety of patients in accordance with non-medical prescribing law. In the clinical scope of practice such as palliative and end-of-life care, there are complex patient presentations caused by the dying and disease process (such as cancer). Such presentations require additional expertise to ensure that standards are maintained and the training principles associated with becoming a non-medical prescriber are adhered to. The NMC order acknowledges that medicines pose a significant risk to patients, which includes our older patient cohort as their pharmaceutical responses differ from adults. This should also be considered in patients who are dying as a large proportion of these patients are 75 years and older. This is to ensure that patients are safe; the prescribing is effective in treating the patients' need and considers cost, but ultimately that NMPs who are specialists in palliative care and possess the skills, knowledge and competence to support those who are in either the last year or the last days of their lives.

## 12.7 Case Studies

In this section of the chapter, I have provided some examples where a specialist palliative care nurse with the non-medical prescribing qualification could benefit patients who are at the end of their lives.

### 12.7.1 Scenario 1

A patient is admitted over the weekend as an outlier onto a surgical ward with a suspected bowel obstruction. Following an urgent CT scan, the surgeons determined that there was no single site of obstruction that could be managed surgically and their care was transferred to the oncology team. The palliative care CNS was working over the weekend and received a referral for symptom management for this patient. On arrival to the ward, the patient was in clear pain and recognised that this admission would be for terminal care and management of symptoms. The palliative care CNS worked collaboratively with the doctors to ensure the patient's symptoms were met; however, due to the nature of a busy surgical ward and weekend junior doctor cover, the patient experienced a delay in the prescription for the syringe driver and anticipatory medications being written. This is suboptimal care for a patient with severe life-ending symptoms, which can lead to patient, family and staff distress.

### 12.7.1.1   The Benefits of NMP

- Immediate prescription of syringe driver and anticipatory medications to assist in alleviating the symptoms of a bowel obstruction: pain, nausea, sickness and agitation
- Reduction of delays in the patient receiving symptom alleviating medication
- Ability to re-review and provide dose adjustments if patients symptoms permit
- Better patient experience

## 12.7.2   Scenario 2

A patient had been referred to the palliative care team and being cared for in the emergency admissions unit. They were being supported by the team for their symptoms associated with their chronic, life-limiting illness. On review and thorough assessment of the patient, there were some changes identified that would warrant changes in the analgesia that the patient was receiving (an increased dose). The palliative care CNS paged the appropriate doctor and documented in the patients' notes regarding the recommendations required to assist in managing the patients' increased pain. The nurse then went the following day to review the patient's pain in light of the increased analgesia. Unfortunately the recommendations had not been performed; therefore, the patient's pain was no better than 24 h previously.

### 12.7.2.1 The Benefits of NMP

- Reduction in delays (in excess of 24 hours) for adjustment to prescriptions being prescribed.
- Patient's pain could have been reassessed, and further dose adjustments or switch in analgesia could have been recommended if the initial changes had been made.
- Increased authority for the nurse to manage the patient's symptoms.
- Alleviation of symptoms for the patient resulting in greater patient experience and confidence in their management.

These scenarios highlight the benefit of nurse prescribers in palliative care, which would ultimately benefit the patients who are dying. The following aspects should also be taken into consideration:

> NMP could lead to reduction in the collaborative working partnerships with palliative care teams and other teams therefore diminishing responsibility for the recognition of symptoms, the deteriorating/dying patient and training of our junior doctors in the management of those who are dying.

## 12.8 Conclusion

In conclusion this chapter has highlighted the key priorities for patients who are in the last days and years of life and the national strategies and frameworks in place to support the patient, their loved ones and staff involved in this important aspect of care delivery. Literature highlights the benefits for patients having access to nurses who possess the non-medical prescribing qualification. The advantages are direct access to symptoms management, and medications being prescribed by those with specialist training and knowledge, which inevitably will improve patient outcomes and experience in achieving a better death.

Whilst acknowledging the above, it is widely accepted that in a specialism such as palliative care, there are numerous constraints that may prevent nurses from prescribing as effectively as the literature sets out. These can include lack of support within the organisation for prescribers, the complex, multifaceted symptoms presented by those who are dying and the use of potential products used outside of the conditions of their product license (off label) medicines for symptoms.

With this in mind and on the whole, patients certainly benefit if nurses who work within specialist palliative care possess a non-medical prescribing qualification.

# References

Andrews A, Morgan G (2012) Constipation management in palliative care: treatments and the potential of independent nurse prescribing. Int J Palliat Nurs 18(1):17–22

Cole T, Gillet K (2015) Are nurse prescribers issuing prescriptions in palliative care? Nurse Prescr 13(2):98–102

Creedon R, O'Regan P (2010) Palliative care, pain control and nursing prescribing. Nurse Prescr 8(6):257–264

Culshaw J, Kendall D, Wilcock A (2013) Off label prescribing in palliative care: a survey of independent prescribers. Palliat Med 27(4):314–319

Dawson S (2013) Evaluation of nurse prescribing in a community palliative care team. Nurse Prescr 11(5):246–249

Department of Health (2008) End of life care strategy: promoting high quality care for all adults at the end of life. Available at https://www.gov.uk/government/uploads/system/uploads/attachment_data/file/136431/End_of_life_strategy.pdf. Accessed 28 Dec 2016

Farrell C, Molassiotis A, Beaver K et al (2011) Exploring the scope of oncology specialist nurses' practice in the UK. Eur J Oncol Nurs 15(2):160–166

Lennan E (2014) Non-medical prescribing of chemotherapy: engaging stakeholders to maximise success? Ecancermedicalscience. doi:10.3332/ecancer.2014.417

National Institute of Clinical Excellence (2004) Guidance on cancer services improving supportive and palliative care for adults with cancer, The manual. Available via https://www.nice.org.uk/guidance/csg4. Accessed 28 Dec 2016

National Institute of Health and Care Excellence. NICE (2015) Care of the dying adult in the last days of life. Available at https://www.nice.org.uk/guidance/ng31. Accessed 15th June 2017

National Palliative and End of Life Partnership (2015) Ambitions for palliative and end of life care: a national framework for local action 2015–2020. Available via http://endoflifecareambitions.org.uk. Accessed 28 Dec 2016

Nursing and Midwifery Council (2006) Standards of proficiency for nurse and midwife prescribers. NMC, London

Nursing and Midwifery Council (2015) The code: professional standards of practice and behaviour for nurses and midwives. NMC, London. Available via https://www.nmc.org.uk/standards/code/. Accessed 28 Dec 2016

Quinn B, Lawrie I (2010) Developing nurse independent prescribing in a specialist palliative care setting. Int J Palliat Nurs 16(8):401–405

Stenner K, Carey N, Courtenay M (2012) Prescribing for pain. How do nurses contribute? J Clin Nurs 21(23–24):3335–3345

The Gold Standards Framework (n.d.) Available via http://www.goldstandardsframework.org.uk. Accessed 28 Dec 2016

Webb WA, Gibson V (2011) Evaluating the impact of nurse independent prescribing in a weekend clinical nurse specialist service. Int J Palliat Nurs 17(11):537–543

Wilson E, Morley H, Brown J et al (2015) Administering anticipatory medications in end-of-life care: a qualitative study of nursing practice in the community and in nursing homes. Palliat Med 29(1):60–70

Ziegler L, Bennett M, Blenkinsopp A et al (2015) Palliative care: a regional survey. Palliat Med 29(2):177–181

# Index

**A**

Accountability, 8, 10, 11, 45, 103, 136–137, 180–181, 187, 206

Acute care, 23, 25

Adherence, 162, 168–171, 173, 207

Advanced nurse practitioner (ANP), 22, 23, 84, 178, 180, 181, 189, 191, 192

Advanced practitioner, 25

Alcohol dependence, 203, 206

Allied health professions, 113–126

Anticipatory medicines, 224

Audit, 43–45, 188, 189

Autonomy, 18, 20, 95


**B**

Barriers to prescribing, 152

*British National Formulary (BNF)*, 19, 25


**C**

Clinical governance, 40, 45–47

Clinical management plan (CMP), 6, 57, 58, 61, 122, 123, 199, 200, 202, 203

Clinical nurse specialists (CNSs), 23, 197, 219, 220, 224–226

Clinical specialist independent non-medical prescribers, 134

Communication, 10, 35, 104, 163, 173, 186–187, 192, 225

Communication Concordance, 168–170

Community, 2, 19, 20, 23–25, 34, 36, 56, 77–79, 81, 82, 95–98, 100, 134, 135, 140–141, 145–156, 191, 197, 220, 223, 225–227

© Springer International Publishing AG 2017
P.M. Franklin (ed.), *Non-medical Prescribing in the United Kingdom*,
DOI 10.1007/978-3-319-53324-7

Community (*cont.*)
  care, 58, 67, 72–74, 84
  nurses, 34, 36, 41, 42
Community practitioner nurse
  prescribing, 4, 7, 9
Concordance, 139, 168–170
Consultation, 10, 36, 39, 56, 61,
  66, 99, 115, 137, 138, 141,
  149, 150, 155, 160, 162,
  164–169, 172, 173, 225
Continuing professional
  development
  (CPD), 10, 45–47
Crown Report, 18
Cumberlege Report, 34

**D**
De-prescribing, 170–173
Devolved country, 35
Dietician, 42
Dispensing, 97, 100, 104, 108
District nurses, 34

**E**
Electronic health records, 134
Electronic Prescribing Analysis
  and Cost (ePACT) data,
  153
End-of-life care (EOLC), 155,
  215–231

**G**
General practice, 43, 44, 76, 81,
  84, 107, 145, 146, 150, 155,
  156
Governance, 70, 72, 75–77,
  79–81

**H**
Health visitors, 34, 36
Hospice, 225–226
Hospital at Night, 178–179

**I**
Independent prescriber, 97,
  98, 103
Independent prescribing,
  115–117, 119–121,
  123–125
Independent prescribing
  supplementary
  prescribing, 5–9

**L**
Liability, 180–181
Long-term condition
  (LTC), 2, 80, 108, 137,
  155–156, 159–173, 203
  management, 80, 108,
  155–156, 163

**M**
Medication Appropriateness
  Index (MAI) tool, 146
Medicines optimisation,
  137–138, 147–149
Minor ailments, 99, 104–107
Mobile working, 149–151
Monitoring, 36, 43–45
Multi-professional, 37, 42,
  146, 156, 165
  training, 37

**N**

National Treatment Agency (NTA), 198, 199
Non-medical prescriber, 19, 20, 23–26
Non-medical prescribing, 1–11, 17–26, 53–85
Northern Ireland, 53–85
*Nurse independent prescriber*, 19
Nurse practitioner, 18, 21
Nurse prescriber, 19
Nurses, 18–21, 23–25, 34, 36–39, 41, 42, 56, 57, 59–63, 66, 72, 76, 77, 84
Nursing, 18, 21, 22

**O**

Optometris, 41, 42
Optometrists, 60, 61, 63–64, 66, 72, 77–80, 84
Outside the product licence, 149

**P**

Pain management, 68, 124, 146, 221
Palliative care, 4, 24, 66, 69, 71, 155, 216, 218–231
Patient care, 4, 10, 22, 34, 48, 84, 94, 133, 149, 150, 160, 186, 187, 192, 219
Patient group direction (PGD), 97, 105, 106, 117, 119, 121, 122, 148, 149, 179, 189, 190
Patient safety, 39, 40, 48, 70, 150, 164, 202

Pharmacists, 36–39, 41, 42, 56–62, 66–77, 79, 81–83, 93–108
Physiotherapists, 41, 42, 59–60, 64–67, 80–81, 85
Physiotherapy, 114, 116–121
Podiatrist, 41, 42
Podiatrists, 59–60, 64–67, 80–81, 85
Podiatry, 114, 116–121, 124
Polypharmacy comorbidities, 203
Prescribing, 53–85
Prescribing of medicines, 35, 36, 39, 41
Prescribing prescriptions, 19, 23
Prescription only medicines order, 40
Primary care, 21, 24, 36, 40, 43, 58, 59, 67, 72–85, 97, 106, 121, 135, 146, 152, 155, 196, 200, 204, 209, 227
Public health, 18, 56, 63, 104, 181, 188, 196, 205, 206, 208–210

**R**

Radiographer, 41, 42
Radiography, 114, 116–117, 120–124
Recovery, 198, 205, 207, 208
Remote prescribing, 182
Repeat prescribing, 35, 36, 97

**S**

Scottish Government, 19–23, 26
Secondary care, 23, 24, 26

Shared care, 186–187, 190,
        192, 200, 208
Shared decision-making, 139,
        169, 223
Specialist community public
        health nurses (SCPHNs),
        151–154
Substance misuse, 195–210
Supplementary prescriber
        Education, 99
Supplementary prescribing, 4, 5,
        9, 35–38, 40, 42, 49, 57–61,
        63, 80, 84, 117, 121, 122,
        200, 202, 204
Supply of medicines and
        Administration of
        medicines, 34, 35

**T**
Therapeutic relationship,
        138–139
Training and support, 217,
        227–228


**U**
United Kingdom, 18–21, 26


**W**
Wales, 33–49